Oral Microbiology at a Glance

DATE DUE

Oral Microbiology at a Glance

Richard J. Lamont

Professor of Oral Microbiology
University of Florida College of Dentistry
USA

Howard F. Jenkinson

Professor of Oral Microbiology
University of Bristol
UK

WILEY-BLACKWELL

A John Wiley & Sons, Ltd., Publication

Blackwell Publishing was acquired by John Wiley & Sons in February 2007. Blackwell's publishing programme has been merged with Wiley's global Scientific, Technical, and Medical business to form Wiley-Blackwell.

Registered office
John Wiley & Sons Ltd, The Atrium, Southern Gate, Chichester, West Sussex, PO19 8SQ, United Kingdom

Editorial offices
9600 Garsington Road, Oxford, OX4 2DQ, United Kingdom
2121 State Avenue, Ames, Iowa 50014-8300, USA

For details of our global editorial offices, for customer services and for information about how to apply for permission to reuse the copyright material in this book please see our website at www.wiley.com/wiley-blackwell.

Library of Congress Cataloging-in-Publication Data
Lamont, Richard J., 1961-
   Oral microbiology at a glance / Richard J. Lamont, Howard F. Jenkinson.
      p. ; cm. — (At a glance series)
   Includes index.
   ISBN 978-0-8138-2892-3 (pbk. : alk. paper)
   1. Mouth—Microbiology—Handbooks, manuals, etc.   I. Jenkinson, Howard F.   II. Title.
III. Series: At a glance series (Oxford, England)
   [DNLM: 1. Mouth—microbiology—Handbooks.   2. Mouth Diseases—microbiology—Handbooks.
3. Tooth Diseases—microbiology—Handbooks. QW 39 L234o 2010]

QR47.L36 2010
617.5′22—dc22
                                                                            2009027990

A catalogue record for this book is available from the British Library.

Set in 9/11.5pt Times by Graphicraft Limited, Hong Kong
Printed and bound in Singapore by Fabulous Printers Pte Ltd

1   2010

Contents

About the authors

Dr Richard J. Lamont is Professor of Oral Microbiology at the University of Florida. He received a PhD from the University of Aberdeen in 1985 and has been studying and teaching oral microbiology ever since. His research interests revolve around the molecular basis of dental plaque development and the cellular interactions between oral bacteria and the host epithelium.

Dr Howard F. Jenkinson is Professor of Oral Microbiology at the University of Bristol, UK. He received a PhD from the University of Nottingham in 1978 and worked on the molecular genetics of *Bacillus subtilis* before embarking on a career in oral microbiology research and teaching. His main research interests involve studies of molecular mechanisms of colonization and pathogenesis by *Streptococcus*, *Candida* and *Treponema*.

Both Drs Lamont and Jenkinson are the recipients of Distinguished Scientist awards from the International Association for Dental Research in recognition of their contributions to oral microbiology.

Preface

This book is designed to provide basic science students, medical students, and especially dental students, with a comprehensive but easily digestible introduction to oral microbiology. We have provided a very short history of the subject because it is not always appreciated that studies on oral bacteria are at the roots of today's microscopy and cultivation techniques. The oral microbiota is very complex in composition, but it is not so important to remember the names of the microorganisms as it is to understand how they collectively contribute to oral disease, and indeed to oral health. Since we are both microbiologists with interests in fundamental molecular mechanisms, we have tried to explain not just what happens, but how it happens. We would like to thank the following colleagues for the provision of images and/or helpful comments on the text: Tom Brown, Karen D'Antuono, Lindsay Dutton, Dave Dymock, Valeria Gordon, Murray Hackett, Erik Hendrickson, Masae Kuboniwa, Gwyneth Lamont, Sarah Maddocks, Ruben Mesia, Angela Nobbs, Helen Petersen, Manfred Rohde, Frank Scannapieco, Luciana Shaddox, Terje Sjöström, Dominic O'Sullivan, Sarah Ellison and Chris Wright.

Richard Lamont
Howard Jenkinson

1 Introduction to oral microbiology

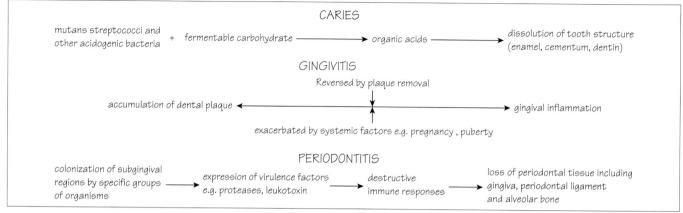

Figure 1.1 Etiology of the major bacterial diseases in the oral cavity

Table 1.1 Important oral diseases, their manifestations and the major microorganisms involved.

Disease	Description	Microorganisms implicated
Caries	Decay (loss) of tooth enamel (dental caries) or dentin (dentinal caries), or root dentin (root aries)	Streptococcus, Lactobacillus, Actinomyces (root caries)
Gingivitis	Redness and swelling (inflammation) of the gingival tissues (gums)	Actinomyces, Fusobacterium, Bacteroides, Prevotella
Periodontitis	Inflammation and either rapid (aggressive, either generalized or localized) or slower (chronic) destruction of the tissues supporting the tooth	Aggregatibacter (localized), Porphyromonas, Treponema, Tannerella, Fusobacterium, Prevotella
Implantitis	Infection and destruction of tissues surrounding a dental titanium implant	Staphylococcus, Pseudomonas, Porphyromonas, Prevotella
Pulpitis	Infection of the pulp, inflammation around the apex of the root, leading to abscess formation (periapical granuloma)	Fusobacterium, Dialister, Peptostreptococcus, Porphyromonas
Halitosis	Oral malodor	Fusobacterium, Porphyromonas, Prevotella, Treponema, Eubacterium
Pharyngitis	Redness and inflammation of the pharynx	Group A Streptococcus, Neisseria, Haemophilus, Coxsackie A virus
Tonsillitis	Infection and inflammation of the tonsils	Group A Streptococcus, Haemophilus
Leukoplakia	White patches on the buccal mucosal epithelium or tongue	Candida, human papilloma virus (HPV)
Stomatitis	Reddening and inflammation of the oral mucosa	Candida albicans, Candida tropicalis, other Candida species
Actinomycosis	Hard swelling (cyst) within the gums	Actinomyces israelii
Cold sores	Surface (superficial) red, dry lesions close to the lips	Herpes simplex virus (HSV)

The oral cavity is the most complex and the most accessible microbial ecosystem of the human body. The teeth, gingivae (gums), tongue, throat and buccal mucosa (cheeks) all provide different surfaces for microbial colonization. The constant production of saliva and intermittent provision of sugars and amino acids from ingested food provides nutrients for microbial growth. The human oral cavity is home to about 700 identified species of bacteria. This number will probably turn out to be closer to 1000 in the future, when all taxa and phyla have been recorded. It is also home to at least 30 species of fungi (mainly of the genus *Candida*), several species of protozoa (which graze on the bacteria for food), and various intracellular viruses. Generalizing, in a single subject it is usual to find between 20–50 species of bacteria at healthy oral sites. At diseased sites there is a tendency for higher numbers of different species to be present, perhaps 200 or more. These facts underline two main features in the field of oral microbiology. There are a number of different micro-environments within the oral cavity and the ecology of these is complex and diverse. Second, microorganisms do not exist as single species; rather they are almost always present in communities.

Commensals and pathogens

The organisms present in the oral cavity are a mixture of commensals and pathogens. A commensal microorganism is defined as one that lives on or within a host but does not cause any apparent disease. However, this terminology may be misleading, as many commensal bacteria can, under certain conditions, be associated with human disease. Subjects whose immune systems are not working optimally, i.e. immunocompromised, are especially susceptible to infections by microbes that are commensal in healthy individuals. For these reasons, commensals are nowadays often referred to as opportunistic pathogens.

Many of the cultivated bacteria present in the mouth probably contribute to oral diseases to a greater or lesser extent, because these diseases are almost always associated with polymicrobial infections (see Figure 1.1). Monospecies infections are rare; however, localized aggressive periodontitis (LAP) is predominantly associated with *Aggregatibacter actinomycetemcomitans*, while *Actinomyces israelii* can cause oral cysts (see Table 1.1). Overt pathogens are organisms that usually cause disease when present, unless the host has protective immunity. There are

very few organisms in the oral cavity and nasopharynx that can be considered overt pathogens. *Streptococcus pyogenes* (Group A Streptococcus), *Streptococcus pneumoniae* (Pneumococcus), *Neisseria meningitidis* (Meningococcccus) and *Haemophilus influenzae* all reside within the nasopharynx and have the potential to cause life-threatening diseases. It is important to note, however, that even in such cases these bacteria may also be carried by subjects with no overt signs of disease. This is termed the carrier state. Vaccination of children against meningococcus (MenC) or *H. influenzae* (Hib) has been very effective in protecting against disease. In addition, the immunization programs have led to reductions in the numbers of carriers of these bacteria in the human population. One of the problems with this kind of approach is that removal of one species of bacteria from a population creates a vacant niche for arrival of other organisms. This might result in replacement by a similar species of different serotype that is not covered by the vaccine. This occurs in children immunized using the 7-serotype (heptavalent) pneumococcal conjugate vaccine. Alternatively, a different bacterium may become resident, such as *Staphylococcus aureus* on the nasal mucosa of subjects immunized against Pneumococcus.

Oral diseases

Almost every member of the human population is afflicted at some stage of their lives with an oral disease (see Table 1.1). The incidence of dental caries has declined generally in the developed world, due in part to fluoride in the water supply, in toothpaste, or taken in tablet form. However there are many groups within societies that are still seriously afflicted with caries. Polymicrobial infections of the gingivae and sub-gingival regions (periodontitis, implantitis and pulpitis) are major conditions requiring clinical intervention. These diseases impose a significant burden on the heath care system. Halitosis is often caused by bacteria on the tongue processing proteins into volatile sulfur compounds. Pharyngitis and tonsillitis are common diseases in children and are caused by bacteria or by viruses (see Table 1.1). Osteonecrosis of the jaw is associated with the use of bisphosphonates particularly in cancer patients with multiple myeloma. Fungal infections, most frequently by the yeast *Candida albicans*, are associated with reduced salivary flow, ill-fitting dentures, hormonal changes, or compromised immune function. Viral infections of the oral mucosa include HPV, EBV and HSV.

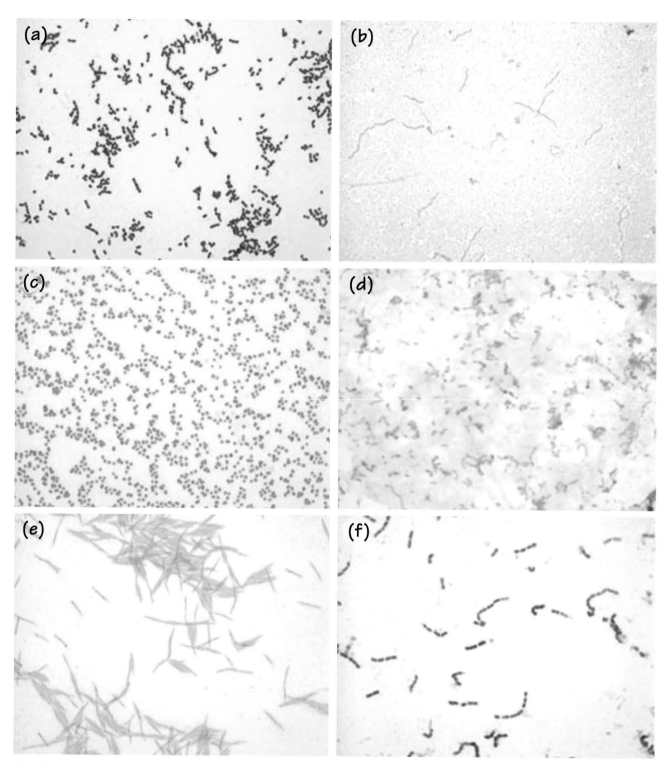

Figure 2.1 Gram stains of important oral bacteria observed by microscopy: (a) Streptococcus gordonii; (b) Treponema denticola; (c) Neisseria sp.; (d) Porphyromonas gingivalis; (e) Fusobacterium nucleatum; (f) Peptostreptococcus micros (Parvimonas micra). Gram-positive bacteria stain purple while Gram-negative bacteria stain pink.

Evidence that humankind has long practiced dentistry comes from archeological findings. The ancient Egyptians, Greeks and Romans produced carefully shaped ivory or bone teeth, sometimes held together with metal wire. In the Middle Ages dentistry was practised by barber-surgeons. Toothache was cured by extraction, with no anesthetic, except perhaps alcohol. By 1800 the scientific study of dentistry was beginning to emerge. The first use of ether as an anesthetic for tooth extraction was in 1846. The growth of dentistry and dental surgery led to the opening of schools, the first in Baltimore (1839) and then a school at the London Dental Hospital, Soho Square, in 1859.

The first microbes

The beginnings of microbiology as a subject lie with oral microbiology. Antoine van Leeuwenhoek was the first recorded scientist to discover microorganisms. He wrote in 1676 about the white stuff between his teeth that, when examined under his extraordinary microscopes with hand-made lenses, contained "animalcules" or little animals. Some of the microbes that he recorded in his drawings may be recognized today as classic bacterial rods, cocci, fusiforms and spirochetes (see Gram stains of these types of organisms in Figure 2.1). However, these detailed studies were not linked to oral disease at that time as tooth decay was thought to originate within the tooth (vital theory). Later, the chemical theory held that putrification of food produced a chemical that dissolved enamel. A microbial etiology for caries began to emerge in the 1840s when Erdl described microorganisms from carious lesions that were proposed to cause decay.

Microbial basis of infectious disease

In the late nineteenth century, Robert Koch discovered the infectious nature of anthrax, the bacterium causing tuberculosis, and the vibrio bacterium that caused cholera. Koch was the first to grow bacterial colonies on gelatine, a solid medium later developed as agar. He described different colony morphologies and concluded that the smaller colonies comprised microbial cells that divided more slowly than those within the larger colonies. However, he is best known for Koch's postulates, which today are still the basis for proving that a disease is caused by a specific microorganism. The postulates are that the microorganism must be: found in all cases of the disease examined; prepared and maintained in pure culture; capable of producing the original infection in animal models; and retrievable from an infected host. The reason that these are introduced here is because many oral diseases are not caused by one microorganism, but by polymicrobial consortia of bacteria. In these cases one bacterium depends upon the presence of others to grow or to express virulence factors. In addition, the human oral microbiota is unique to humans; therefore few appropriate animal models are available to fulfill Koch's postulates for oral diseases. This means that Koch's postulates must be modified for the unique oral situation and combine information from studies of association, treatment, host responses and virulence factors.

Miller and the chemoparasitic theory of caries

WD Miller, an American microbiologist working in Berlin, laid the foundation of modern oral microbiology. Miller was able to observe oral bacteria within tissues, in particular streptococci penetrating the tubules of dentin. Miller's most significant contribution was to synthesize the work of Koch (isolation of pure cultures), Pasteur (fermentation of sugars to lactic acid) and Magitot (fermentation of sugars could dissolve teeth *in vitro*), and to expand the theories of Mills and Underwood, to formulate the chemoparasitic theory (1890). In essence correct, this theory states that caries is caused by acids produced by oral bacteria following fermentation of sugars. With the description of dental plaque independently by Black and by Williams in 1898, the key elements of our modern concept of the etiology of dental caries were in place. It is noteworthy, however, that it was not until the mid-1970s that there was a consensus view that periodontal disease (periodontitis) is caused by oral bacteria.

Oral and dental research

With the establishment of dental schools and oral biology/microbiology departments in the USA and UK, came research and new developments in dental microbiology. Dentistry started to become recognized as a science as well as a clinical profession. However, oral microbiology was relatively slow to develop in comparison to other microbiology fields. This was partly because many of the oral microorganisms are anaerobic and require special cultivation methods that were not available at that time. Oral microbiology research was reinvigorated in the USA in 1948, with the establishment of a research facility at the National Institutes of Health, Maryland, which led to the discovery of dental caries as an infectious disease (Chapter 3).

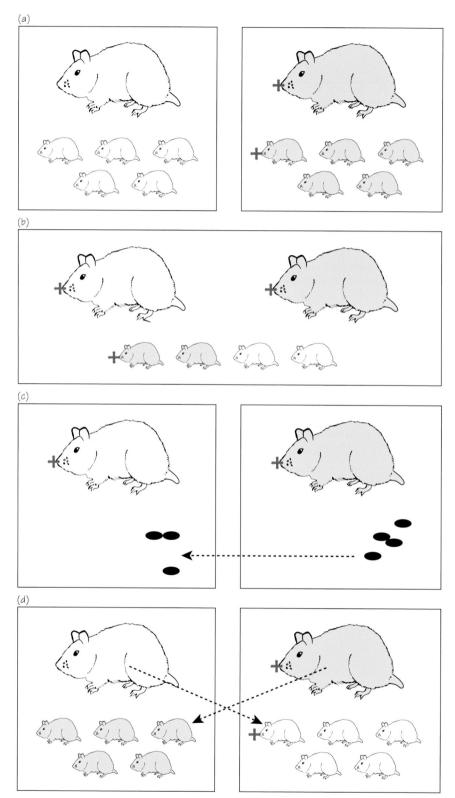

Figure 3.1 Experiments of Keyes and Fitzgerald in the 1950s to test whether caries was an infectious or genetically determined disease using golden or albino hamsters and their pups. **+** Indicates the presence of caries. Redrawn with permission from Slots J, Taubman MA (eds) *Contemporary Oral Microbiology and Immunology* (1992), Mosby Year Book, St Louis.

In 1920s London there were several groups of microbiologists studying various aspects of human infections. Killian Clarke worked at the Royal Dental School, where research was funded only through charitable contributions. Clarke researched in collaboration with Fish at St Mary's Hospital, Paddington, where four years later Fleming discovered penicillin. Clarke described a spherical bacterium that formed chains of cells, isolated from dental caries lesions. He named this organism *Streptococcus* (streptus (Greek) flexible chain, and coccus (Greek) berry) *mutans* (different morphological forms which he believed were mutants). *S. mutans* produced lactic acid as a main by-product from glucose fermentation (homolactic). But there was a strong cohort of *Lactobacillus* microbiologists at the time, and Clarke's attempts to have *Streptococcus* named as a new genus were foiled. With the depression of the 1930s and the outbreak of the Second World War, this discovery was not followed up in the UK.

Dental caries as a transmissible disease

The National Institutes of Health, Bethesda, USA, established a dental research institute in 1948. Fitzgerald and Keyes had set up a germ-free animal unit, and noted that a line of golden hamsters developed tooth decay when fed a high sugar diet, while an albino line of hamsters did not (see Figure 3.1a). Either tooth decay was genetic, or the golden hamsters carried an agent that the albinos did not. To demonstrate that caries was due to an infectious agent, a series of novel and exacting experiments were undertaken. When the two lines of hamsters were caged together, all adult females and their pups developed dental caries (panel b). The fecal pellets from the golden hamsters, when transferred to the albinos, resulted in the albinos developing caries (c). Lastly, caries-free albino pups, when transferred to a golden hamster mother, went on to develop caries (d). These observations suggested that caries was a transmissible disease, and not a genetic condition.

Streptococcus mutans

By the late 1950s, Keyes and Fitzgerald began working on the nature of this transmissible factor. A *Streptococcus* was purified from carious lesions of hamsters (also from rats) that was strongly acidogenic (producing acid) and non-proteolytic. When these bacteria were fed to *Streptococcus* and caries-free hamsters, dental caries then developed in those animals on a high sugar diet. The *Streptococcus* could be recovered from the mouths of infected hamsters, and shown to cause caries when re-inoculated into germ-free animals. These observations fully satisfied Koch's postulates. Interestingly, it turned out that the albino hamsters were only caries free because they had been exposed to high concentrations of antibiotics in previous studies aimed at establishing germ-free animals. It was not until 1968 that it was accepted that the *Streptococcus* isolated from hamsters was the same *S. mutans* as that described by Clarke in 1924.

Mutans group streptococci

Following this pioneering work with hamsters and rats, many laboratories throughout the world, along with the NIH group, went on to isolate *S. mutans*-like bacteria from humans and monkeys. These bacteria were shown to induce dental caries in hamsters, rats, gerbils and monkeys. The organism *S. mutans* is now subdivided into species including *S. cricetus* (hamster), *S. rattus* (rat), *S. ferus*, *S. macacae* (monkey), *S. sobrinus*, and *S. downeii*. These are referred to as the mutans group streptococci.

Link between *S. mutans* and dental caries

Further studies with animals led to a temporal relationship being established between colonization by mutans group streptococci and subsequent attack on the teeth to generate white spot (early caries) lesions. Epidemiological studies in humans then began to seek correlations between numbers of *S. mutans* present on teeth and the development of dental caries. Numerous studies suggested positive correlations, and so led to the idea that *S. mutans* levels were a good indicator of active caries, and may indeed be predictive. Strip or dip culture methods were developed to monitor mutans group streptococci levels in saliva samples from children. High levels of mutans group streptococci often correlated well with caries activity in populations. However, these correlations were not perfect and often broke down at the level of individual patients. Today it is clear that there are individuals and population groups of high caries susceptibility with low levels of mutans group streptococci and vice versa. The reasons for these remain largely unexplained.

Immunity to caries

Because dental caries resulted from bacterial infection, this led to ideas that immunity could be induced. Immunization against dental caries in primates was reported in 1969. Since then many studies have demonstrated that serum antibodies, mainly immunoglobulin G (IgG), and salivary antibodies, mainly secretory immunoglobulin (S-IgA), are induced following vaccination of animals with *S. mutans* cells or purified *S. mutans* antigens. Development of a vaccine for humans has not yet occurred (see Chapter 21), and even if scientifically achievable may not be accepted for what is (most commonly) not a life-threatening disease.

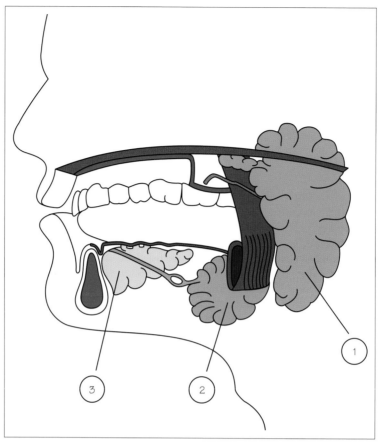

Figure 4.1 Positions of the major salivary glands (1 parotid; 2 sub-mandibular; 3 sub-lingual).

Table 4.1 Major functions of saliva.

1 Physico-mechanical flushing
2 Tissue coating: lubrication and permeability barrier
3 Modulation of the oral microbiota
4 Antacid and neutralization of deleterious materials
5 Regulation of calcium and phosphate equilibrium
6 Digestion

Table 4.2 Major components of salivary pellicle.

Albumin
Amylase
Lysozyme
Lactoferrin
Acidic proline-rich proteins
Proline-rich glycoproteins
Statherin
Mucin-glycoprotein (MG)1
MG2
Carbonic anhydrase
Secretory immunoglobulin A (S-IgA)

Around 0.5 to 1.5 liters of saliva are secreted into the mouth each day. Saliva is responsible for flushing the epithelial surfaces and for lubrication and protection of tissues, and an adequate flow of saliva is essential for the maintenance of both hard and soft tissue integrity. Saliva is hypotonic, with an average pH of around 6.7. Saliva contains both organic compounds (2–3 g/l protein, notably the enzyme amylase) and inorganic compounds including the electrolytes bicarbonate, chloride, potassium and sodium.

Most of the important physiological properties of saliva have been deduced from subjects who have deficiencies in saliva flow rate, saliva production, or in specific salivary components (Table 4.1). Salivary flow rate and composition can be affected by a range of infectious diseases, clinical conditions, e.g. wearing of dentures, clinical treatments, e.g. radiation therapies for oral cancer, or pharmaceutical drugs. The symptoms of dry mouth (xerostomia), due to deficiencies in salivary flow, are frequently accompanied by increased susceptibility to oral microbial diseases as is discussed in the following chapters.

Saliva production

There are three pairs of salivary glands in the human (see Figure 4.1). The parotid glands (shown as (1) in Figure 4.1), with the parotid ducts emanating in the cheeks, supply a fluid containing bicarbonate and phosphate ions, agglutinins (glycoproteins), α-amylase (degrades starch), proline-rich proteins and a range of other proteins and glycoproteins. Plasma cells, originating in the bone marrow, localize to the parotid glands and produce S-IgA which is also present in parotid secretions. The sub-mandibular glands (2) located beneath the floor of the mouth, produce about 70% of saliva in the oral cavity, and this contains mucous and serous (serum derived) components. The sub-lingual glands (3) located anterior to the sub-mandibular glands produce mainly mucous secretions. There are many other minor salivary glands located throughout the oral cavity. Von Ebner's glands are found in the papillae of the tongue, and they produce a serous secretion that is essential for taste. It is suggested that because whole saliva contains serous proteins (derived from gingival crevicular fluid), as well as body cells (from tissues in the mouth), it may in the future provide a means for more rapid diagnosis of conditions that currently require blood or tissue samples for analysis.

Protective role of saliva

There are between 1 million and 100 million bacteria present in 1 ml of saliva, depending upon oral hygiene, frequency of food consumption, and salivary flow rate. Saliva in the fluid phase acts principally to flush out bacteria from the mouth. Saliva contains agglutinins that aggregate bacteria, thus preventing adherence to surfaces, and the bacterial clumps are removed by swallowing or expectoration (Chapter 5). Saliva possesses a number of additional antimicrobial components that are discussed in the succeeding chapters.

Salivary pellicle

Saliva forms a coating on all the surfaces that are present in the mouth, and at the back of the throat. Teeth, gums, dentures, mouth guards, all get rapidly coated with salivary components. A thick mucus coating forms on the soft tissues. The mucus concentrates the many hundreds of different proteins, glycoproteins, glycolipids and lipids present in saliva so they form a protective film. The salivary films formed on hard surfaces, such as natural teeth, or dentures, are very thin (less than 1 micron) and are known as acquired pellicle (Table 4.2). Acquired pellicle on enamel forms around 30 seconds after eruption of the tooth or professional cleaning. The composition of the acquired pellicle differs according to the surface on which it is formed. Enamel is ionic in composition and so binds to charged molecules. Acrylic materials used in denture production can be hydrophobic and lack significant electrostatic charge, so bind to molecules that are uncharged.

Components that are released from bacterial and host cells can also be incorporated into pellicle. Transglutaminase from epithelial cells can be found in pellicle. GTF and FTF (Chapter 16) from bacteria can become incorporated into pellicle and remain enzymatically active, thus increasing the levels of the associated glucan and fructan polymers. In that regard, amylase in pellicle remains active and may continue to hydrolyze starch to glucose that can be used by oral streptococci for fermentation with resultant acid production.

The acquired pellicle provides receptors for bacterial adhesion. For example, the agglutinins that aggregate bacteria in suspension also promote adhesion when deposited in the enamel pellicle. Interestingly, some salivary molecules, such as the PRPs, will only bind bacteria when deposited on surfaces, as a conformational change in the protein occurs which exposes previously hidden binding sites (cryptitopes). Proteolytic activity by some organisms such as *P. gingivalis* can also expose cryptitopes. Fortunately, as bacteria and their hosts have co-evolved, the organisms that bind to immobilized salivary components on surfaces tend to be oral commensals. Unrestricted plaque build up, however, will irritate the gums and cause inflammation (gingivitis).

Saliva as a nutrient

Saliva can provide growth nutrients for bacteria. Various bacteria produce proteases that degrade salivary proteins into peptides and amino acids, which can be used by the bacteria when exogenous nutrients are limiting. Bacteria can also produce glycan hydrolases that cleave sugar residues from the salivary glycoproteins, so that the sugars can be used for bacterial growth. Again, through co-evolution the bacteria that readily colonize and grow in saliva are mostly harmless and may help exclude pathogens.

5 Salivary mucins and agglutinins

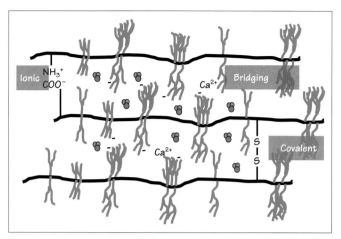

Figure 5.1 Mucins are the basis of saliva function. Alignment of mucin chains by ionic or covalent bonds, or by calcium ion bridging, traps water to form a hydrated gel.

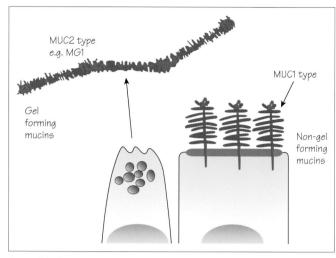

Figure 5.2 Gel forming and membrane bound mucins in the oral cavity.

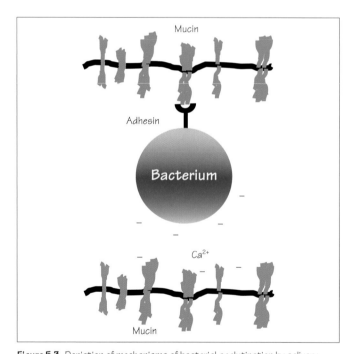

Figure 5.3 Depiction of mechanisms of bacterial agglutination by salivary mucins, involving direct interaction of bacterial surface proteins with mucin carbohydrate chains, and Ca^{2+} bridging of negative charges.

Table 5.1 Characteristics of mucins.

Large extracellular molecules with many sugar chains

Membrane bound or gel-forming

Mucin domains rich in serine, threonine, proline

Oligosaccharides (glycans) linked to hydroxy amino acids via N-acetyl-galactosamine

Site-specific, e.g. salivary mucins different from intestinal mucins

Mucins are present at all surfaces within the human body that are exposed to the environment. The outer layers of mucosal surfaces are comprised of epithelial cells. These can be highly keratinized (such as in the nose or insides of the cheeks), less keratinized (gums), or ciliated (respiratory tract). Salivary mucins are extremely large proteins carrying chains of sugar residues linked together. The permutations of sugar linkage, in linear or branched structures, are almost endless, hence the study of mucin biology is very complex. In saliva there are two main types of mucin, designated mucin glycoprotein 1 (MG1) and the smaller mucin glycoprotein 2 (MG2). MG1 is encoded by the *MUC5B* gene and MG2 is encoded by the *MUC7* gene. Mucins are produced by all salivary glands except (or in very low amounts) by the parotid gland.

Composition of mucins

Mucins are composed of an amino acid chain backbone (polypeptide) with chains of sugar residues attached to the amino acids serine, threonine, or asparagine (Table 5.1). The sugar chains (oligosaccharides) may be spread all over the molecule or localized to specific regions. The most frequently found saccharides are sialic acid (N-acetylneuraminic acid, NeuNAc), glucose (Glc), galactose (Gal), fucose (Fuc), N-acetyl-glucosamine (GlcNAc), N-acetyl-galactosamine (GalNAc), and mannose (Man). The oligosaccharide chains and the amino acids work in conjunction to determine the biochemical properties of mucins.

Properties of mucins

Mucins form complexes that are key to their functional properties. Charged carboxyl or amino groups present on amino acids can form ionic cross links with oppositely charged groups on adjacent polypeptide chains. Cysteine residues present in one chain can form disulfide bonds with cysteine residues in another chain. Both of these inter-chain interactions tend to align mucin chains with each other (Figure 5.1). Sialic acid residues, which are highly negatively charged, can then interact with sialic acid residues on aligned chains through bridging with Ca^{2+} ions. The sialic acid residues are very important to mucin function, as they are to other systems in the human body. The negatively charged residues act to keep the mucin chains apart, allowing water molecules to become trapped between them. Mucin function depends upon this trapping of water molecules, thus determining the degree of hydration of the mucin gel. Mucin has high viscosity when it is hydrated and gel-like, and MG1 is the main gel-forming mucin in saliva (Figure 5.2). The viscosity and elastic properties of saliva are attributed to the gel-forming mucins. These have multiple cysteine-rich domains that form disulfide bonds and thus generate multimeric complexes. The non gel-forming mucins provide a relatively close coating of epithelial cells, protecting the cell membrane from physical or biological damage. Some of them are membrane tethered (Figure 5.2). They lack the cysteine rich domains of the gel forming mucins.

Bacterial agglutination

Since bacteria usually have a net negative surface charge, they tend not to bind directly to negatively charged mucins. Instead, they may interact through bridging reactions involving divalent cations such as Ca^{2+} ions (see Figure 5.3). However, many bacteria express cell surface proteins (lectins) that specifically recognize oligosaccharides present on the salivary mucins. In this manner salivary mucins are bound by multiple bacteria and agglutination results. MG2 is thought to be more important than MG1 for agglutinating bacteria in saliva. Agglutination of some oral streptococci is lost after removal of the terminal sialic acid of the oligosaccharide side chains, indicating that the bacterial lectin has sialic acid specificity. Another high molecular weight agglutinin is the parotid glycoprotein gp340 (also known as salivary agglutinin, or DMBT1), a member of the scavenger receptor cysteine-rich protein family. gp340 agglutinates *S. mutans* cells through Ca^{2+}-dependent interaction with an alanine rich repetitive domain of the AgI/II family P1 protein on the streptococcal surface. gp340 also agglutinates group A streptococci and the N-terminal cysteine rich domain of gp340 interacts with HIV gp120 sequences and inhibits viral infection. Other salivary compounds that can aggregate bacteria include lysozyme, β_2-microglobin and S-IgA (Chapter 6). As mentioned in Chapter 4, agglutinins that are present in the acquired pellicle on enamel surfaces can act as receptors for bacterial adhesion and promote colonization.

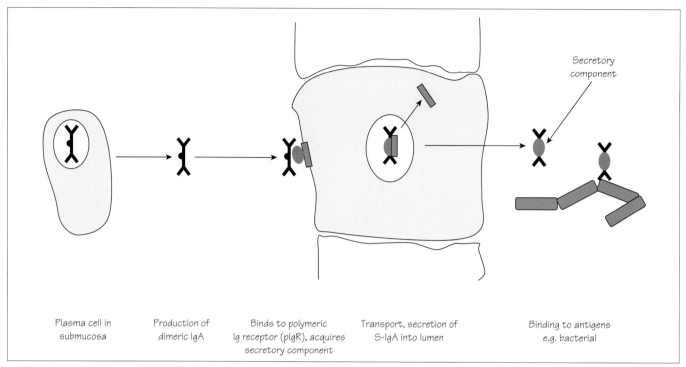

Figure 6.1 Steps in production and secretion of IgA at the mucosal surface.

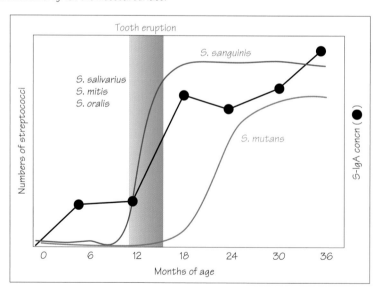

Figure 6.2 Graph depicting the time of acquisition of different streptococci in the mouth after birth, and the development of the secretory immune system after one year, approximately coincident with tooth eruption.

Table 6.1 Acquisition of oral immune functions.

Age (months)	Antibody (source and type)
0–6	Maternal IgG (serum)
	Maternal IgA (milk)
12–18	Infant IgG (teething)
18–36	Infant IgA (saliva)

The major immunoglobulin in the salivary secretions is immunoglobulin A (IgA). This molecule is secreted as a complex with a linking chain by cells that are found close to the parotid gland. The secreted form of IgA is called secretory IgA (or S-IgA). It is found at all mucosal sites, such as the gastrointestinal tract, respiratory tract and urogenital tract, and it is also present in tears and breast milk (in addition to saliva). There are two isoforms, or subclasses, of IgA designated IgA1 and IgA2 and saliva contains approximately equal proportions of each. IgA is also found in serum (where IgA1 is in higher concentration) and is made by bone marrow B cells. In the blood, IgA interacts with a receptor on immune effector cells designated CD89. This initiates inflammatory reactions and activates phagocytosis by macrophages. IgA1 recognizes protein antigens whereas IgA2 is directed against polysaccharides, LPS and LTA. IgA is found in secretions as S-IgA, which consists of two (dimeric) or four (tetrameric) IgA monomers held together by a joining chain (J chain) polypeptide, and by a secretory component (SC) polypeptide.

Production of S-IgA

Polymeric IgA (mainly the secretory dimer) is produced by plasma cells in the lamina propria which is found underlying mucosal surfaces. Polymeric IgA binds to the polymeric immunoglobulin (Ig) receptor protein (pIgR) present on the basolateral surface of epithelial cells and is taken up into the cells by endocytosis. The receptor-IgA complex traverses the cellular compartments and is secreted at the luminal (outside) surface of the epithelial cells still attached to the receptor. The pIgR receptor is then cleaved by protease and the dimeric IgA molecule, linked by the J chain, and containing a portion (SC) of pIgR, are free to diffuse into the secretions (Figure 6.1).

Functions of S-IgA

The primary function of S-IgA is immune exclusion. S-IgA is glycosylated and this anchors S-IgA to the mucus lining of the epithelial surface and thus inhibits attachment and tissue penetration by viruses, bacteria, and their released antigens such as LPS, toxins and environmental antigens. IgA antibodies do not activate complement, thus minimizing disruption of the epithelial barrier layer. Free in saliva, polymeric IgA effectively aggregates bacteria. Glycans on S-IgA are also able to non-specifically trap bacteria. S-IgA interacts with mucins and so-called scavenger proteins such as gp340 present in saliva to generate heterotypic complexes that trap bacteria and stimulate macrophage migration.

Inactivation of salivary defenses

The oral microbiota has evolved to grow and survive in the human mouth despite the salivary defenses, and these organisms have devised means to resist IgA and salivary defenses. For example, some *Streptococcus*, *Haemophilus* and *Neisseria* species produce proteases that specifically cleave S-IgA1, disrupting functions such as complexing and clumping. S-IgA1 fragments may also promote bacterial adherence and accumulation. IgA2 has a deletion in the hinge region that renders it resistant to these proteases. Other bacteria produce glycan hydrolysases that cleave sugar chains from mucins. This causes changes in mucin properties making them much less efficient, both in binding bacteria and in lubrication.

Development of S-IgA

At birth, a child has a poorly functioning immune system. Serum antibodies are mainly derived from the mother, and the child produces no S-IgA antibodies. It takes over a year to generate a significant salivary IgA titer (see Figure 6.2). Colostrum and breast milk are rich in S-IgA antibodies so it is thought that these provide protection against oral, oropharyngeal and GI tract infections in children. The main source of immune protection for a child up to 12 months is thus from the mother (Table 6.1).

The window of infectivity

After about six months of age, the first teeth begin to erupt. This is associated with a change in the oral microbiota to incorporate bacteria that adhere well and colonize the tooth surfaces. While *Streptococcus salivarius* and *Streptococcus oralis* are already colonizing the oral mucosal surfaces, when teeth start to appear bacteria such as *Streptococcus sanguinis* and *Streptococcus mutans* are provided with a hard surface to colonize (Figure 6.2). The main agent of dental caries, *S. mutans*, tends to appear later in the mouth than *S. sanguinis*, and follows an increase in IgA titer. This so-called window of infectivity (Figure 6.2) may be important for the oral health of the child. It has been found that the earlier children acquire *S. mutans* then the greater their risk of childhood caries.

Selective IgA deficiency

This is a genetic immunodeficiency in which the serum level of IgA is undetectable, although levels of the other main immunoglobulins IgG and IgM are normal. Although the amount of IgA produced is similar to the total of all other Igs combined, IgA deficiency is largely asymptomatic. This is most likely because IgM can compensate for IgA, and those individuals that are also defective in IgM have a higher caries incidence. IgA deficiency also causes a slight increased risk of oral, respiratory and gastrointestinal infections, and of developing autoimmune diseases in middle age.

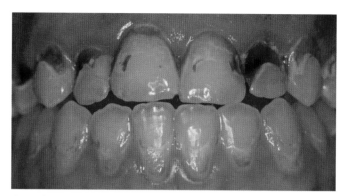

Figure 7.1 Rampant caries such as occurs in patients with xerostomia (reduced salivary flow).

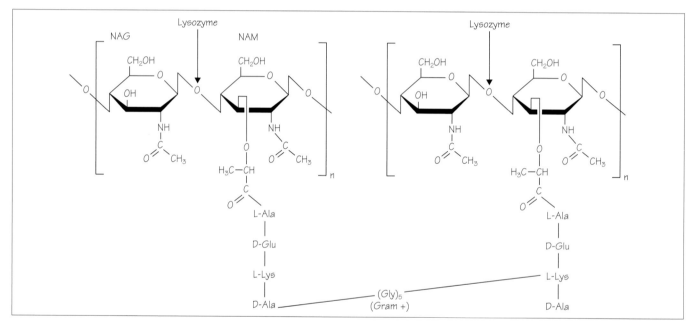

Figure 7.2 Action of lysozyme on Gram-positive bacterial peptidoglycan which consists of repeating units two joined amino sugars, N-acetylglucosamine (NAG) and N-acetylmuramic acid (NAM), with a pentapeptide coming off of the NAM. Lysozyme cleaves the β-(1,4)-glycosidic bonds.

Table 7.1 Properties of salivary histatins that inhibit oral bacteria and fungi.

Family of histidine rich peptides in saliva
Histatin 5 potent inhibitor of *Candida albicans*
Does not work like the HBDs
Binds to receptor, peptide enters the cells, cell cycle arrested, efflux of ATP, respiratory apparatus inhibited
Anaerobic cells are less susceptible

Impaired salivary flow is deleterious to oral health. For example, an inadequate salivary flow rate increases the incidence of dental caries (see Figure 7.1), for at least three reasons. First, there is greater bacterial retention in the mouth and more dental plaque forms; second, the acids produced by bacteria such as mutans group streptococci are inefficiently neutralized; and third, the enamel surface does not efficiently re-mineralize.

Agglutination, physical flushing of bacterial and salivary IgA are discussed in the preceding chapters; however, saliva also contains a number of anti-microbial compounds that can restrict plaque accumulation and kill bacteria and other microorganisms.

Anti-microbial components in saliva

(1) Lysozyme Lysozyme is a basic protein found in most secretions, including saliva, where it is present in high concentrations. Salivary lysozyme originates from both the salivary gland secretions and from gingival crevicular fluid (GCF). Lysozyme digests the cell walls of Gram-positive bacteria by breaking the β(1-4) bond between *N*-acetylmuramic acid and *N*-acetylglucosamine in peptidoglycan (Figure 7.2). Lysozyme can also activate autolysins in bacterial cell walls. Not surprisingly, many successful oral colonizers are relatively resistant to killing by lysozyme. Lysozyme can also bind and aggregate bacteria and facilitate clearance by swallowing or expectoration. In addition, lysozyme contains small amphipathic sequences in the C-terminal region that are capable of killing bacteria.

(2) Salivary peroxidase Peroxidase in saliva is derived from the salivary glands and PMNs, and catalyzes the oxidation of thiocyanate (SCN^-) to hypothiocyanite ($OSCN^-$) by hydrogen peroxide, which is produced by the aerobic metabolism of oral bacteria. At acid pH, $OSCN^-$ becomes protonated (and uncharged) and readily passes through bacterial membranes. Hypothiocyanite oxidizes SH groups in bacterial enzymes and inhibits bacterial metabolism. Reduction of hydrogen peroxide to water by peroxidase also prevents oxidative damage to the host soft tissues.

(3) Lactoferrin Lactoferrin is an iron binding glycoprotein produced from glandular acinar cells, epithelial cells and phagocytic cells.

Lactoferrin inhibits bacterial growth by binding and sequestering Fe^{2+} ions, and in the apo (iron free) state can be toxic to bacteria and interfere with bacterial adhesion. A 25-residue N-terminal proteolytically derived peptide fragment termed lactoferricin also kills bacteria through depolarization of cytoplasmic membranes.

(4) Histatins Histatins are cationic histidine rich proteins that kill *Candida albicans* and some bacteria (Table 7.1). At least 12 histatins are present in saliva, resulting from truncations or proteolysis of the genetically distinct histatins 1 and 3. Histatin 5 (the N-terminal 24 amino acids of histatin 3) is a major salivary histatin and is very effective in killing yeast. Histatins bind to a *Candida* membrane receptor, then the peptide is taken up by the cells. This results in arrest of the cell cycle and the cells lose ATP by efflux. Histatins can also regulate hydroxyapatite crystal growth, inhibit bacterial cysteine proteinases and prevent bacterial coaggregation.

(5) Cystatins Cystatins are cysteine rich peptides that inhibit bacterial cysteine proteases. Cystatins also regulate inflammation by inhibiting host proteases and up-regulating cytokines. Von Ebner gland protein is another cysteine protease inhibitor.

(6) Chromogranin A Chromogranin A is produced by the sub-mandibular and sub-lingual glands, and is processed to release an N-terminal peptide, vasostatin-1, which is antibacterial and antifungal.

(7) Antiviral factors These include secretory leukocyte protease inhibitor (SLPI), gp340, Thrombospondin 1 (TSP1) and proline rich proteins (PRPs). SLPI is a serine protease inhibitor that can inhibit the infectivity of the HIV virus, and is also bactericidal and fungicidal. TSP1 is a high molecular weight extracellular matrix glycoprotein that is secreted by the sub-mandibular and sub-lingual glands. TSP1 can bind to regions of the HIV gp120 protein and prevent binding to CD4. Basic PRPs may also inhibit HIV infectivity by binding to gp120.

Salivary glands also produce β-defensins (Chapter 8), and whole saliva will contain serous proteins derived from the gingival crevicular fluid (GCF, Chapter 9) and compounds released by epithelial cells. Hence, whole saliva contains low levels of IgG, IgM and complement components from GCF, and calprotectin (a calcium binding anti-microbial protein) from epithelial cells.

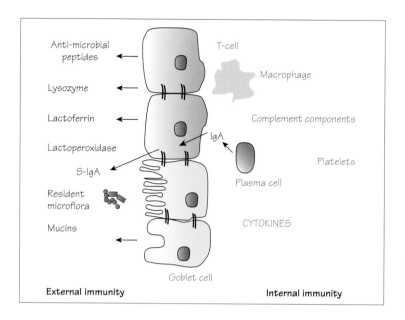

Figure 8.1 Major components of the innate defense system. Redrawn with permission from Henderson B, Wilson M, McNab R and Lax A (eds) *Cellular Microbiology* (1999), John Wiley & Sons, Chichester.

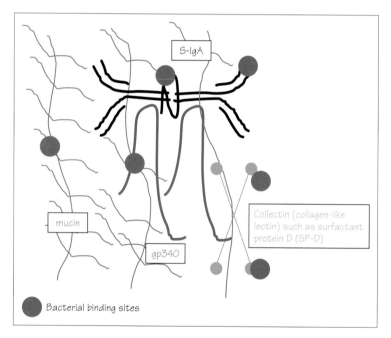

Figure 8.2 Multiple salivary molecules possess binding sites for bacteria that can facilitate entrapment of organisms and clearance.

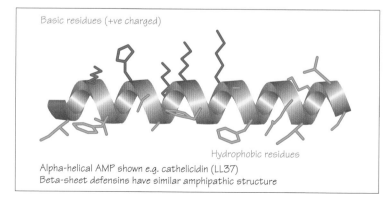

Figure 8.3 Amphipathic structure of anti-microbial peptides (AMPs).

Innate immunity is non-specific and does not require prior exposure to infectious agents, so it is "always on". In the oral cavity, the first layer of innate immunity comprises physical barriers such as the epithelium; phagocytic cells such as polymorphonuclear neutrophils (PMNs) that are recruited from the circulation into the gingival tissue and the sub-gingival region; and inhibitory actions of commensal microorganisms (Figure 8.1). In addition, the oral fluids possess anti-microbial factors as discussed in Chapter 7, many of which can bind and entrap microorganisms (Figure 8.2). The second line of innate immunity is inflammation that acts to localize infectious agents at sites of mucosal penetration. Inflammation also provides a link between innate immunity and acquired immunity.

Epithelial and phagocytic cells utilize pattern recognition receptors (PRRs) such as Toll-like receptors (TLRS) to bind and characterize microbe associated molecular patterns (MAMPs), repeating patterns of molecules not found on host cells. Examples of MAMPs include LPS of Gram-negative bacteria, LTA of Gram-positive bacteria, peptidoglycan, flagellin, pilin, unmethylated CpG islands of bacterial DNA, fungal mannans and viral double-stranded DNA. There are at least 11 TLRs that recognize distinct MAMPs. TLR binding to a MAMP signals epithelial cells and leukocytes to secrete proinflammatory cytokines and chemokines, and anti-microbial peptides through activation of the transcription factor NF-κB.

Within the cytoplasm of leukocytes and epithelial cells, the NOD (nucleotide binding oligomerization domain)-like receptor family recognize MAMPs derived from intracellular bacteria and also activate proinflammatory cytokines and anti-microbial peptides through NF-κB. NOD1 recognizes a specific peptidoglycan fragment containing diaminopimelic acid, more frequently found in Gram-negative bacteria. NOD2 recognizes a muramyl dipeptide (MDP) fragment derived from peptidoglycan which is common to both Gram-positive and Gram-negative bacteria. Other NOD-like receptors (NLRs) can detect dsRNA and dsDNA. Upon detection of specific MAMPs, some NLRs undergo conformational changes and assemble a molecular platform called the inflammasome. The inflammasome processes and activates pro-caspase 1 and the resultant active enzyme mediates proteolytic maturation of the inflammatory cytokines IL-1β and IL-18.

As both commensal and pathogenic organisms express MAMPs that will be recognized by TLRs and NLRs, activation of an inflammatory response may also require the participation of so-called "danger signals" released by dying or injured cells, which indicate the presence of pathogenic activity.

Epithelial cells and leukocytes produce nitric oxide which is a free radical that is toxic to bacteria by causing DNA damage and degrading of iron sulfur centers into iron ions and iron-nitrosyl compounds.

Anti-microbial peptides (AMPs)

These are natural antibiotics produced by insects, shellfish, frogs, toads, mammals, etc. There are many different classes, but most peptides contain between 20 and 40 amino acid residues. The sequences of these peptides are different but their properties are similar. They adopt amphiphilic (or amphipathic) architecture, one side being positively charged and the other side being hydrophobic (Figure 8.3). The positively charged side interacts directly with biological membranes, and this then helps the molecule enter the membrane and form pores which leads to membrane disruption. AMP activity depends principally upon the lipid composition of the membrane, and mammalian cells that express specific AMPs are rendered resistant to their action by virtue of a lower phospholipid composition. AMPs may be useful antibiotics in the future, particularly as AMPs are even active against methicillin resistant *Staphylococcus aureus* (MRSA) and work in seconds on susceptible bacteria. While AMPs have a broad spectrum of activity, some bacteria are resistant. For example, *Salmonella* is resistant to macrophage AMPs. Also, *S. aureus* cells produce modified membrane lipids or wall teichoic acids that resist binding of the positively charged AMPs. *P. gingivalis* becomes more resistant to AMPs following exposure to environmental stresses, including sublethal doses of β-defensins. Less pathogenic members of the oral microbiota such as some *F. nucleatum* strains are inherently resistant to the action of AMPs in the oral cavity. Biologically active AMPs cannot be chemically synthesized at present, so there is much interest in trying to find the minimal active portions and synthesize these commercially.

Human AMPs

Defensins, produced by humans and primates, are 15 to 20 amino acid residue peptides with six to eight conserved cysteines. The alpha-defensins in humans (six known to date) are produced by leukocytes, PMNs and intestinal Paneth cells. The beta-defensins are produced by epithelial cells and leukocytes. There are four major types (HBD1-4) and many other variants. HBD1 is expressed constitutively in oral epithelial cells, while HBD2 is induced by bacterial infection. Cathelicidin LL37 is produced by leukocytes, skin and respiratory epithelia. These proteins are all important in protecting against microbial infections, particularly when the acquired immune system is in the development stages. However, AMPs are not just anti-microbial, they cause histamine release from mast cells, interact with complement, are chemotactic for monocytes, enhance wound closure, stimulate antigen-presenting dendritic cells and stimulate cytokine production. Moreover, HBD3 induces expression of the costimulatory molecules CD80, CD86 and CD4 on monocytes and myeloid dendritic cells in a TLR-dependent manner.

9 Microbes in the oral cavity

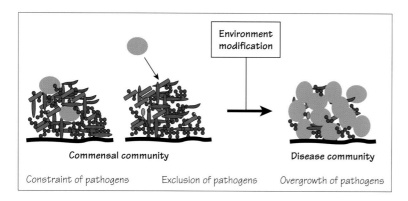

Figure 9.1 *Depiction of commensal and pathogenic microbial communities. In commensal communities, pathogens (blue) can be present but constrained or excluded by the commensals. The right panel reflects the ecological plaque hypothesis whereby conditions change such that pathogens can become dominant.*

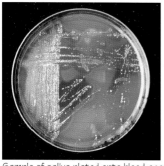

Complex microenvironment
with multiple host influences

Two major outcomes for bacteria

A stable bacterial community
working towards the common
good

or

Intense competition between
bacterial communities

Sample of saliva plated onto blood agar, multiple colony types, some hemolysis (clearing) and some discoloration (browning) of the blood due to Fe^{3+} and hydrogen peroxide production.

Figure 9.2 *Opposing constraints in the colonization of the oral cavity.*

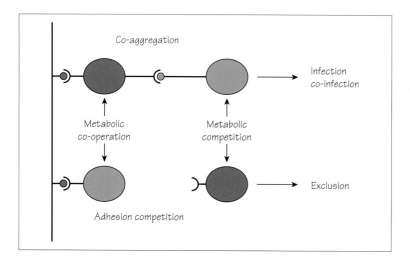

Figure 9.3 *Synergistic and antagonistic interactions among oral bacterial colonizers. Commensal (blue) and potentially pathogenic (purple) bacteria might coexist in oral microbial communities. Provided that the pathogen can use available receptors for adhesion, either on the host surface or on the surfaces of antecedent bound bacteria, and provided that metabolic deficiencies or dependencies are fulfilled, the pathogen grows and survives in the microbial community. Depending upon host susceptibility this could potentially result in a polymicrobial infection typical of most oral diseases. In the lower half of the diagram, the combined effect of receptor unavailability and nutritional inadequacy, either because the necessary partner organisms are not present or because the environment is unfavorable, leads to exclusion of the potential pathogen from the community. Reproduced with permission from Jenkinson HF, Lamont RJ Oral microbial communities in sickness and in health. Trends in Microbiology (2005): 13, 589–595.*

Table 9.1 Colonization or invasive disease?

Continuous interplay between microbes and host

Bacteria respond rapidly to host environmental changes

Microbial communities are self-limiting

Bacteria compete for adhesion receptors

Virulence factors prolong intracellular survival and promote tissue damage

Many of the bacteria present in the oral cavity are anaerobic (growing only in the absence of oxygen under reduced conditions) or facultatively anaerobic (able to grow under more oxidized conditions, but also anaerobically). The anaerobic organisms are able to grow and survive because of the presence of the facultative anaerobes and aerobic (oxygen-requiring) bacteria. These facultative and aerobic bacteria remove oxygen and oxidized compounds from the environment and thus generate conditions that are oxygen depleted and reduced. The bacteria that initially colonize the salivary pellicle on the tooth surface, tongue, palate and pharynx are mainly facultative anaerobes. Most of the bacteria within the genus *Streptococcus* fall into this category, as do many of the other microbial species associated with coronal plaque, including plaque formed within fissures of the tooth crown. In addition, the fungus *Candida albicans* is facultatively anaerobic and can tolerate low pH. Candida is able to colonize the buccal epithelium and the tongue, but can also be found in carious lesions where the pH is < 5.0.

Primary colonizers

Bacteria that first colonize salivary pellicle present on the tooth surface are designated primary colonizers, and are mainly streptococci. The major species include *Streptococcus oralis*, *mitis*, *sanguinis*, *parasanguinis* and *gordonii*. In addition, *Actinomyces*, *Veillonella*, *Gemella*, *Abiotrophia*, and *Granulicatella* are usually detected. These bacteria, except *Veillonella*, stain Gram-positive and are facultative anaerobes. Some of them are difficult to culture in the laboratory, e.g. *Gemella*, *Abiotrophia* and *Granulicatella*. Up to 80% of the organisms present within initial plaque formed on cleaned tooth surfaces are streptococci. Bacterial colonization of mucosal surfaces is less abundant than the tooth surfaces as epithelial cells are continually dying and sloughing off. Communities of bacteria can also survive and develop within epithelial cells without causing host cell death.

Beneficial effects of bacterial colonizers

Despite extensive microbial colonization of many mucosal surfaces, health is the normal state of the host. In the GI tract resident bacteria can be beneficial through a number of mechanisms: (1) provision of simplified carbohydrates, amino acids and vitamins; (2) prevention of overgrowth or colonization of pathogens by competition for niches or nutrients, or by inducing immune cross-reactivity; (3) stimulation of vascularisation and development of intestinal villi; (4) enhancement of the immune system development. These mechanisms are less well studied in the oral cavity; however, resident bacteria can stimulate host innate immune competence. Moreover, oral bacteria induce global changes in the host epithelial cell transcriptome (the pattern of expressed genes, Chapter 11), and these mRNA responses are distinctive for individual organisms.

Ecological plaque hypothesis

Oral disease occurs when the host microbe balance is disrupted at the cellular or molecular level (Table 9.1). Many oral diseases are polymicrobial in origin and both microbial and host factors contribute to the initiation and progression of disease (Figure 9.1). The ecological plaque hypothesis holds that shifts in the relative proportions of organisms can be the forerunner to the development of disease. These populational shifts can be caused by a change in environmental conditions, perhaps caused by dietary intake, or by local or systemic host immune status. As the bacterial community matures, the constituents can cooperate synergistically or be antagonistic to one another (Figure 9.2). The newly dominant bacteria then modify the micro-environment, thus sustaining their presence at the expense of other microorganisms (Figure 9.3).

Ecology and disease

(1) Caries The development of acidogenic plaque containing higher levels of mutans group streptococci able to tolerate lower pH, is promoted by the more frequent dietary intake of fermentable sugars. The rapid increase in the proportions of acid-tolerating bacteria then leads to exclusion of other more acid-sensitive microorganisms.

(2) Gingivitis Inflammation and reddening of the gums (gingivitis) is caused by build up of supragingival plaque at the gingival margins (the line between tooth and gum) and can be exacerbated by calculus (tartar) which is a tissue irritant. Pregnancy, diabetes mellitus and the onset of puberty increase the risk of gingivitis, all associated with hormonal changes that affect host susceptibility. Moreover, many of the oral Gram-negative anaerobes can also metabolize human hormones. The risk of gingivitis is also increased with misaligned teeth, rough edges of fillings and ill fitting or unclean dentures. The sudden onset of gingivitis in a normal, healthy person may be related to viral infection. The inflammation associated with gingivitis is reversible but may, over time, predispose to periodontitis.

(3) Periodontitis This is a long-term chronic condition. Left undisturbed, supragingival plaque will extend down below the gingival margin and become subgingival plaque. The subgingival region between the tooth root and the sulcular epithelium is known as the gingival crevice or sulcus (that deepens to the periodontal pocket in periodontitis). This environment is less oxygenated, which will favor the growth of the anaerobes that can cause periodontal tissue destruction and bone loss. Saliva does not penetrate this region well, and the fluid phase comprises gingival crevicular fluid (GCF). GCF is a serum exudate that contains most serum components, which also favors the growth of oral Gram-negative anaerobes. GCF flow increases with inflammation and will also contain components released from phagocytic cells and epithelial cells.

10 Molecular microbial taxonomy

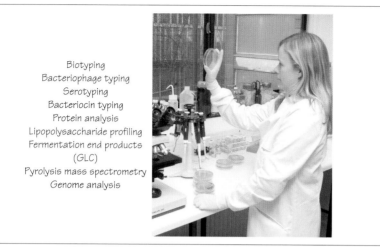

Biotyping
Bacteriophage typing
Serotyping
Bacteriocin typing
Protein analysis
Lipopolysaccharide profiling
Fermentation end products
(GLC)
Pyrolysis mass spectrometry
Genome analysis

Figure 10.1 Techniques used in the identification and subtyping of pure cultures of bacteria.

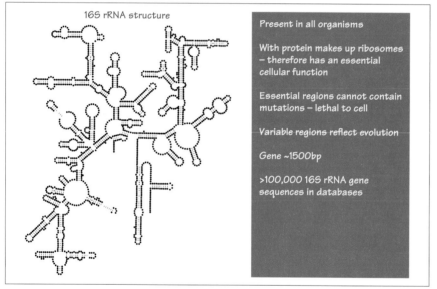

16S rRNA structure

Present in all organisms

With protein makes up ribosomes – therefore has an essential cellular function

Essential regions cannot contain mutations – lethal to cell

Variable regions reflect evolution

Gene ~1500bp

>100,000 16S rRNA gene sequences in databases

Figure 10.2 Features of 16S rRNA.

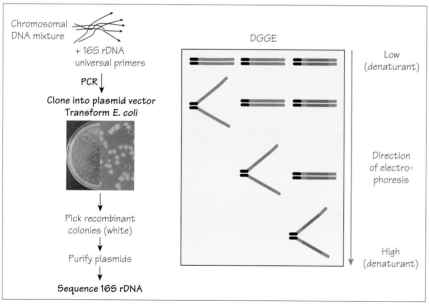

Chromosomal DNA mixture

+ 16S rDNA universal primers

PCR

Clone into plasmid vector
Transform E. coli

Pick recombinant colonies (white)

Purify plasmids

Sequence 16S rDNA

DGGE

Low (denaturant)

Direction of electro-phoresis

High (denaturant)

Figure 10.3 Generalized method for producing 16S rDNA sequence information by PCR-cloning (left panel). Right panel, diagrammatic representation of DGGE (Denaturing Gradient Gel Electrophoresis).

Oral microbiology has traditionally relied on the ability to cultivate bacteria from saliva and from dental plaque in order to define the species present. Originally, only a few species of bacteria were considered of importance in oral disease. However, as culture methods became more sophisticated, particularly with the development of anaerobic cabinets for cultivation of oxygen-sensitive organisms, it became evident that the complexity of microbial species present had been under-estimated. Then, with the development over the last ten years of non-culture molecular methods to identify bacteria, it has become apparent that laboratory cultivation of bacteria alone is inadequate for assessing the complexities of microbial populations. Nowadays, molecular techniques provide sensitive and accurate means to determine snapshots of the microorganisms present, dead or alive, in microbial communities at different oral sites. In addition, there are a number of techniques for the identification of species and subtyping of species into biologically relevant groups or clones (Figure 10.1). Metagenomics describes the study of microbial populations through analyses of the total genomes present. It is important to note, however, that these techniques do not necessarily permit a quantitative measure of the relative numbers of microbes within a community. Other analytical methods such as proteomics, which potentially identifies all proteins present within a sample, may be applied to provide a measure of the functional diversity within a population. A newer technique of metabolomics seeks to identify all the metabolites, by mass spectrometry or NMR spectroscopy, associated with a microbial population. These techniques all aim to provide genetic or biochemical fingerprints of microbial populations so as to relate these to the types of organisms present and, perhaps more importantly, attempt to define patterns associated with diseased sites as opposed to healthy sites.

Molecular taxonomy

As a result of utilizing molecular methods to determine the genomic components of oral microbial communities it is estimated that 40–50% of the oral microbial population is not yet cultivable. This is because the culture media available are not suitable for growing these organisms. In addition, it is likely many grow together as dependent partners or groups and so may be impossible to isolate in pure culture. Molecular methods of identification do not necessarily pick up such dependencies but provide vital information about the microbes present. Molecular taxonomy is generally based around differences in sequences of 16S ribosomal RNA genes (approximately 1500 base pairs) (Figure 10.2). These are present in all microorganisms and together with ribosomal proteins make up the smaller ribosomal sub-unit, essential for protein synthesis. The essential regions within 16S rRNA cannot contain mutations because these are lethal to the cell. However, the variable regions within the genes reflect evolution. There are now > 100,000 16S rRNA gene sequences in databases. Polymerase chain reaction (PCR) is used to amplify the 16S rRNA gene with universal primers that bind to the conserved (essential) regions. The sequence of the gene is then compared with the sequences present in the databases. A > 98% match with a sequence suggests the bacterium belongs to that species. A match of 97% or less indicates a new species or phylotype. To determine the species present in a population, total DNA is extracted, subjected to PCR, and then the rDNA products are cloned and sequenced (see Figure 10.3 left panel).

Denaturing gradient gel electrophoresis

This technique is becoming more popular as a means to identify components within complex microbial population. In this technique PCR amplification across a variable sequence within the rDNA is performed using a primer with a GC-clamp (see Figure 10.2 right panel). The amplicons (approx. 190 bp) are then separated by electrophoresis through a gel with a low to high denaturation gradient of urea and temperature. Those PCR fragments (termed amplimers) with lower GC content (overall fewer H bonds linking the DNA strands) will denature at lower temperature and become retarded within the gel, while those with higher GC content will run further. The GC clamp keeps the amplimer together as double stranded DNA. The separate gel bands are excised, cloned and then sequenced for identification.

DNA chips

With the advent of precise molecular printing techniques, whereby multiple species-specific 16S rRNA gene fragments or oligonucleotides can be imprinted onto membranes or glass slides, it is possible to obtain estimations of bacteria within a population. The analytical power of these kinds of techniques depends entirely upon the accuracy of the information on the DNA chip. In simplest form, plaque or periodontal samples are taken, the DNA extracted, and the 16S rRNA genes for all the bacteria present PCR amplified with fluorescently-labeled universal primers. The amplified material is then hybridized to the DNA from target bacteria present on the chip, and the signal measured from the fluorescent label. Semi-quantitative estimates of numbers of bacteria of interest may be obtained, but only for the 16S rRNA genes of those bacteria which are represented on the chip. More analytically complex, but fundamentally the same, techniques such as checkerboard hybridization, can give multiple comparative readouts of species in different samples.

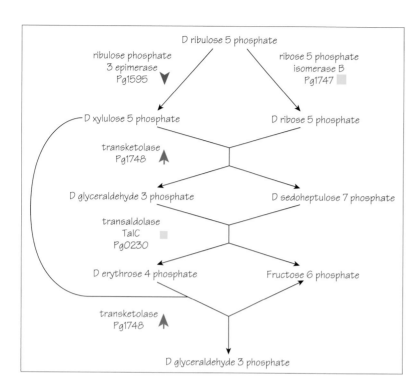

Figure 11.1 Example of ontology for *P. gingivalis* showing the pentose phosphate (non-oxidative) pathway populated from a differential expression proteomics experiment and showing protein abundance changes. Proteins catalyzing each step in the pathway are shown by their *P. gingivalis* gene designation number and protein name. Green downward arrows indicate decreased abundance. Red upward arrows indicate increased abundance. Yellow squares indicate no abundance change.

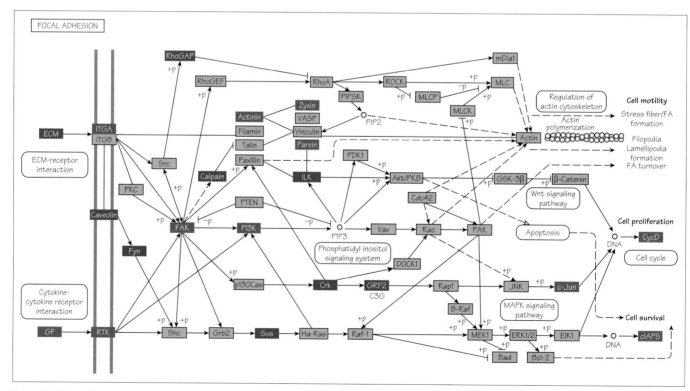

Figure 11.2 Example of ontology for host cell biological pathways involved in focal adhesion. Pathway populated from a differential expression transcriptomics experiment using a microarray to measure mRNA levels in human epithelial cells following challenge with *P. gingivalis*. Red boxes indicate elevated expression and blue boxes indicate reduced expression. Green boxes indicate no expression change.

As the complete genome sequences of oral bacteria are becoming available for an increasing number of organisms, it is now possible to explore bacterial processes such as pathogenicity on a global scale. Genomic sequence can be mined for genes or proteins that are differentially expressed under conditions relevant to disease, such as during infection in humans or in experimental animals, or in *in vitro* models. Genes expressed, up-regulated or otherwise involved in growth or survival under these conditions are candidates for virulence determinants; targets for vaccines or novel therapeutic agents; or have potential for use as diagnostic tools. A number of genome-wide approaches are available, the so called 'omics' disciplines.

Transcriptomics

Transcriptomics is the measurement of the levels of all mRNAs expressed under a particular condition. The transcriptome thus reflects all genes being expressed at a given time. Currently, transcriptomics is usually accomplished using high-throughput techniques based on DNA microarray technology. Microarrays contain spots of DNA target sequence from all genes of the organism. Several unique regions of each gene are amplified or synthesized and attached to a solid support such as a glass slide. RNA is isolated from the organism of interest. Usually the experimental design is to culture the organism under two different conditions. Fluorescently labeled cDNA is prepared from each RNA population, with different fluorescent dyes (usually Cy3 and Cy5) applied in order to distinguish the RNA populations. The labeled cDNA populations are mixed and hybridized to the slide which is then scanned for fluorescent signal intensity attached to the target spots. The strength of fluorescent signal then reflects the level of gene expression.

Proteomics

There is not always a good correlation between the levels of mRNA and the amount of the corresponding protein. As proteins are the major effector molecules of the bacterial cell, measurement of proteins can provide a more accurate view of physiological and metabolic status. Early techniques separated proteins by electrophoresis (either 1D or 2D), and then proteins were identified by sequencing. However, these techniques lacked sensitivity. Currently, the most sensitive technique is to separate whole bacterial lysates into fractions by high pressure liquid chromatography and then feed these fractions directly into a mass spectrometer for protein sequencing. Two bacterial populations can be compared by the differential labeling of one set of proteins with ^{13}C, ^{15}N or ^{18}O which causes a mass offset easily detectable by mass spectrometry.

Mass spectrometry also allows the identification of post-translational modifications of proteins, which often dictate protein activity.

Gene ontology

The predictive power of regulation of individual genes/proteins is limited due to the extensive interconnectivity among bacterial physiological and regulatory networks, and functional redundancy (more than one protein being able to accomplish the same task). Thus, the assembly of regulated genes/proteins into biologically relevant pathways has greater biological resolution. The process of population of pathways with regulated components is known as gene ontology. Successful ontology requires information regarding metabolic and regulatory pathways of the organism under investigation. Such databases are now becoming available for oral bacteria (Figure 11.1). As these pathways become better defined it is possible to predict the system-wide effect of up or down-regulation of any bacterial protein, which then can be confirmed experimentally. For an opportunistic pathogen such as *P. gingivalis*, these approaches hold much promise for further elucidation of pathophysiology and mechanisms of virulence. Human pathway databases can be used to examine host responses to bacteria on a global scale (Figure 11.2).

Post-translational networks

Metabolomics is the comparative, non-targeted analysis of the complete set of metabolites (small organic molecules) in a cell. The power of the metabolome is that it directly reflects the physiological status of a cell. The metabolome is diverse and is continually changing, making it difficult to measure. However, high throughput chromatography and mass spectrometry can provide comprehensive datasets. The interactome is the complete set of molecular interactions in a cell. Examples include protein-protein interactions (the protein interaction network, PIN) or the protein-DNA interactome (important in gene regulation). Other 'omes' being established to provide global information about bacterial cells include the lipidome (total lipids) and the glycome (total carbohydrates).

Tiled arrays

Investigation of regulatory networks is facilitated by the use of tiled arrays. Rather than limiting targets to ORFs (as in conventional microarrays), tiled arrays contain overlapping sequences from the complete genome sequence, which allows identification of elements that bind to regulatory (non-coding) sequences.

12 Oral streptococci

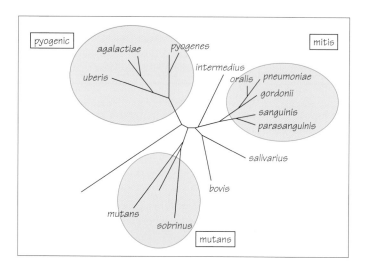

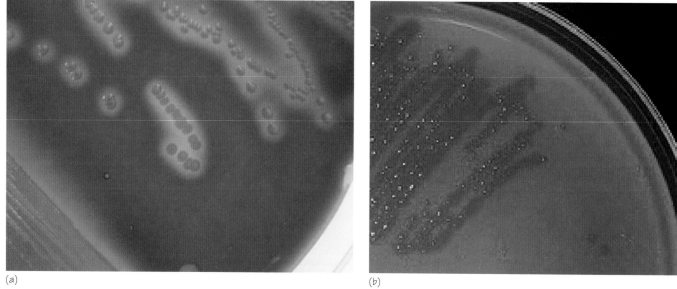

Figure 12.1 *Relatedness within three of the major groupings of streptococci. Adapted with permission from Whiley RA, Beighton D Current classification of the oral streptococci.* Oral Microbiology and Immunology *(1998): 13, 195–216.*

(a)

(b)

Figure 12.2 *(a) Group A streptococci on blood agar showing beta hemolysis. (b) Viridans streptococci on blood agar showing alpha hemolysis.*

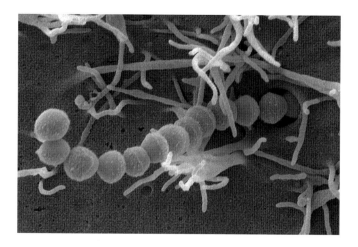

Figure 12.3 *Streptococcus pyogenes interacting with the surface of epithelial cells. The cell membrane forms projections that entwine the bacteria, while uptake of the streptococcal cells occurs through caveolae formation (specific endocytic vesicles lined with the protein caveolin).*

The first oral microorganisms to be cultivated were *Streptococcus mutans* and *Lactobacillus*. These organisms are amongst the family collectively designated as lactic acid bacteria. The group includes the mutans group streptococci, some other oral streptococci (although not all streptococci), and the genus *Leuconostoc*. Lactic acid bacteria characteristically ferment sugars through the glycolytic pathway to form pyruvate, which is then converted to lactate (lactic acid). The amounts of lactic acid produced by the individual bacteria depend upon the environmental conditions, e.g. pH, oxygen. They also depend upon the complement of enzymes present within the bacteria that produce alternative fermentation end products, like acetate (acetic acid), butyrate, propionate and ethanol. The genus *Lactobacillus* contains organisms that are highly acidogenic. This means that they produce large amounts of acid and, as a result, they are also aciduric (meaning able to survive, and sometimes grow, at very low pH). The lactic acid bacteria are characteristically associated with the fermentation of milk, and the generation of fermented milk products, e.g. cheese, yogurt, etc. There is a theory, therefore, that these organisms evolved alongside the emergence of mammals.

The genus *Streptococcus*

Over one hundred species of *Streptococcus* are recognized. Of these, about 50% may be found at some time within the human mouth. Almost all streptococci species are associated with animal hosts, including primates, ruminants, rodents and fish. Interestingly, dogs do not normally carry oral streptococci. Although there are many clear species designations of *Streptococcus*, the individual strains within a species are often very divergent in genotype and phenotype. This is because there is a high frequency of gene transfer between or across the different streptococci. The preponderance for horizontal gene transfer results in a genetic spectrum across the genus *Streptococcus*. Therefore, as more molecular information is obtained from genetic studies, it becomes harder to define individual species within the genus. There is so much variability within the species *S. mitis* and *S. oralis*, which are early colonizers of the teeth and oral mucosa, that individual strains might represent new species in classic terminology. In general though, the human-colonizing *Streptococcus* may be classified into three families: pyogenic (pathogenic), mitis (commensals and pathogens) and mutans streptococci (see Figure 12.1).

Viridans streptococci

The classical name for the oral streptococci is the viridans group. Species of viridans streptococci include *Streptococcus anginosus, gordonii, intermedius, sanguinis, parasanguinis* and the mutans group streptococci. The terminology comes from the observations that many of the oral streptococcal colonies produce a green to brown halo when grown on blood agar. The greening is termed alpha-hemolysis and is a result of the bacteria excreting hydrogen peroxide (H_2O_2) as a by-product of metabolism (Figure 12.2). Oxygen, and other oxidative products, e.g. superoxide ions, which are harmful to the bacteria, are converted to H_2O_2, which then oxidizes the heme present within hemoglobin to form green to brown pigments. In contrast, pathogenic streptococci, e.g. *Streptococcus pyogenes*, produce beta-hemolysis on blood agar. This is exhibited as complete clearing around colonies, caused by lysis of the red blood cells by cytotoxins (Figure 12.2). In *S. pyogenes* these toxins are streptolysin S and streptolysin O.

Lancefield grouping

Many species of streptococci can be assigned to the Lancefield grouping system, pioneered by Rebecca Lancefield at the Rockefeller Institute, New York, from 1929. The Lancefield grouping system depends on a panel of antibodies that react specifically with different carbohydrate antigens present within the cell wall of streptococci. The groups comprise A, B, C, D, E, F, G, H, K, L and R/S. Some of the viridans group streptococci can be Lancefield typed, e.g. *S. mutans* (F), *S. sanguinis* (H), *S. salivarius* (K), but some strains within these species, and *S. pneumoniae*, do not type and are referred to as non-Lancefield type organisms. *S. pyogenes* is a group A *Streptococcus* (GAS). *S. agalactiae* is a group B *Streptococcus* (GBS). GAS strains are further serotyped according to their surface fibrillar M protein. This is anti-phagocytic (protects against phagocytosis) and there are over 150 M types now recognized.

Relatedness and pathogenicity of streptococci

Although it is probably most convenient to use the pyogenic, mitis and mutans groupings, this simplifies a very complex genus. The pyogenic organisms are intracellularly invasive (Figure 12.3), cause invasive diseases and are responsible for pharyngitis, tonsillitis, rheumatic heart disease, acute glomerulonephritis, necrotizing fasciitis (GAS) and neonatal (newborn) infections (GBS). *S. pneumoniae* (also termed pneumococcus) causes serious lung infections (pneumonia) and meningitis, and is responsible for most childhood middle ear infections (otitis media). The mutans group organisms cause dental caries, but when they get into the bloodstream they may also cause infective endocarditis (Chapter 31). The mitis group organisms (but not *S. pneumoniae*) are generally very efficient colonizers of the oral cavity. They orchestrate the development of plaque and so contribute to subsequent development of caries, gingivitis and periodontal diseases.

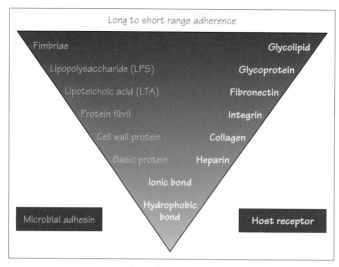

Figure 13.1 Examples of microbial adhesins recognizing host receptors at different ranges.

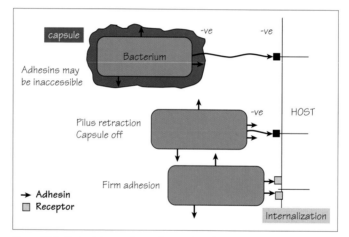

Figure 13.2 Bacterial appendages that mediate long-range adherence and functional consequences of their action.

Table 13.1 Long through short-range adherence.

Host receptor	Adhesin	Microorganism
Glycolipid	Fimbrial (type 1)	Escherichia coli
Glycoprotein	Lipopolysaccharide (LPS)	Pseud. aeruginosa
β_1 Integrin	Hemagglutinin (Fha)	Bordetella pertussis
Fibronectin	Lipoteichoic acid (LTA)	Strep. pyogenes
CEACAM (CD66)	Opa	N. meningitidis
Fibronectin	PrtF(Sfb)	S. pyogenes
Fibrinogen	ClfA	Staph. aureus
Heparin	Basic protein (HlpA)	Streptococcus spp.
Bound Ca^{2+}	Electrostatic (-ve)	Strep. sanguinis
Hydrophobic	Hydrophobic	Candida albicans

Most natural environments in which bacteria exist are open flow systems. This means that to grow and survive under such conditions bacteria must adhere to surfaces and form microbial communities (biofilms). Adherence specificity, together with metabolic processes, determines the ability of a microorganism to colonize an animal host. In the oral cavity, successful colonizers must resist the flushing action of salivary flow together with the mechanical shearing forces of the tongue and lips. Adherence is a potential target for novel therapeutics designed to inhibit bacterial colonization. Infections of catheters, hip replacement joints, contact lenses, dental implants and dentures are major problems that are inadequately controlled by antibiotics and could benefit from such an approach.

Adherence

Bacteria colonize different sites in the human body because they express specific adhesins (usually proteins) (Figure 13.1). These recognize complementary or cognate receptors, often sugars or oligosaccharides, present at different sites. Thus, the buccal mucosal surface comprised of keratinized epithelial cells expresses different receptors from, for example, those present in salivary pellicle. The requirement for a specific complementary receptor to be engaged by a microbial adhesin imparts specificity of bacterial adherence and colonization. Following the initial adherence processes, bacteria will only grow and survive if the immediate chemical environment, e.g. pH, oxygen levels and redox potential, is conducive. It is important to note that adherence is a dynamic process. It is advantageous for bacteria to detach from a surface if the growth conditions are, or become, unfavorable. Consequently, microorganisms have evolved methods for detachment as well as attachment.

Long-range adherence

Bacteria first localize at sites that are thermodynamically favorable. This involves overcoming the repulsive forces that occur between negatively charged surfaces (bacterial and host). One means to accomplish this is through surface appendages such as fimbriae (or pili), which are made up of multiple protein sub-units (polymeric). These extended structures allow for long-range adhesion (across 1 μm or more) to occur. Non-covalent forces such as van der Waals forces, along with electrostatic (if there are positively charged amino acids exposed in the fibrillar proteins) and hydrophobic attraction mediate this adhesion. As the bacterial and host surfaces become closer, hydrogen bonding and divalent cation bridges can also stabilize the interaction (Table 13.1). The combined strength of these bonds can be sufficient for bacteria to remain at a surface long enough to form interbacterial linkages and to allow penetration of the mucous or slime layers present on the surfaces of tissues.

Specific adhesion

Long-range adhesive forces are sufficient for initial attachment but lack specificity, and bacteria can be easily dislodged from the surface. Higher affinity adhesion is provided by complementary adhesins and receptors that fit together much as in an antibody-antigen interaction. Adhesins may be proteins or carbohydrates linked directly to the cell surface, or components of surface structures, e.g. fimbriae that are projected away from the confines of the cell wall (Table 13.1) (Figure 13.2). The protein sub-units of fimbriae (pili) may themselves mediate adherence, or carry the adhesins along their lengths and at their tips. Specificity of microbial adhesion is often associated with protein-carbohydrate (lectin-like) reactions involving specific oligosaccharide receptors. Many microbial adhesins recognize galactose or sialic acid carbohydrate chains or oligosaccharides. However, protein receptors are also common.

Oral bacterial adhesins and receptors

Oral streptococci often possess multiple adhesins which will both increase the affinity of binding and the range of substrates available. Examples, many of which are conserved across species, include (adhesin-receptor): AgI/II family-gp340 and collagen; glucan binding proteins (GBPs)-glucan; AbpA/B-amylase; Hsa-NeuNAc; FbpA-fibronectin. Fibrils on *S. gordonii* (CshA/B-fibronctein) and *S. parasanguinis* (Fap1 protein) also mediate adhesion. *Actinomyces naeslundii* type 1 fimbriae adhere to proline rich proteins (PRPs) present in salivary pellicle, while type II fimbriae attach to sugar residues on epithelial cells. *Porphyromonas gingivalis* long fimbriae (FimA) adhere to PRPs and to salivary statherin in pellicle, as well as directly to host epithelial cell integrins. The *tad* (tight adherence) locus of *Aggregatibacter actinomycetemcomitans* includes genes for the biogenesis of Flp pili, which are necessary for bacterial adhesion to surfaces. Another *A. actinomycetemcomitans* adhesion is Ema, a non-fimbrial protein that binds to collagen. Surface protein adhesin-receptors of other periodontally relevant bacteria include: *Fusobacterium nucleatum* FadA-epithelial cells; *Treponema denticola* Msp-matrix proteins; *Tannerella forsythia* BspA-host cells and matrix proteins. Bacterial surface polymers containing saccharides can also mediate or promote adhesion. Lipoteichoic acids are thought to assist adherence of these bacteria to surfaces. They may operate by ensuring correct presentation of protein adhesins towards their receptors. Polysaccharides that contain sialic acid may promote adhesion of bacteria to human cells, and the LPS of *A. actinomycetemcomitans* is involved in adherence. Adherence processes lead to several possible outcomes: colonization, superficial infection of tissues, intracellular invasion or systemic spread of bacteria throughout the body. Moreover, specific co-adhesion among bacterial species drives the development of the dental plaque community (see Chapter 14).

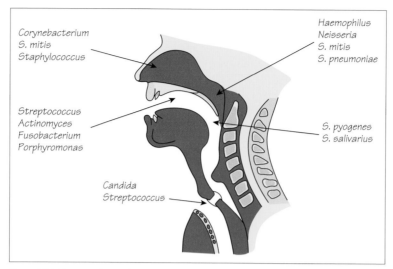

Figure 14.1 Site specificity of microbial adherence and colonization.

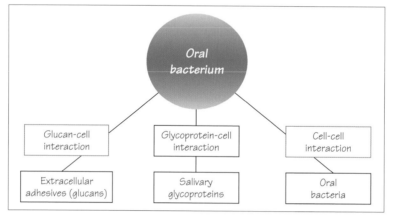

Figure 14.2 Major adherence mechanisms of oral bacteria.

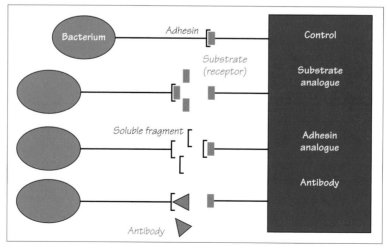

Figure 14.3 Strategies to inhibit bacterial adhesion.

Specificity of adhesion (Chapter 13), along with environmental constraints arising from host and other bacterial influences, imparts specificity to microbial colonization patterns (Figure 14.1). The first stages of dental plaque formation, already discussed, involve the attachment of bacteria to salivary proteins and glycoproteins that are deposited as pellicle on the surfaces of teeth and other hard surfaces (like dentures). The pioneering bacteria are *Streptococcus, Gemella, Granulicatella* and *Actinomyces*. As they build up on surfaces so they form the base layers for the development of complex dental plaque biofilms. Complex plaque begins to develop on a clean tooth surface after 4–6 hours. Plaque develops more quickly at the gingival margins where salivary flow forces are lower, and the micro-environment is more protected.

Inter-microbial reactions

The development of plaque is an ordered, temporal sequence of events, rather than random coming together of different bacteria. The primary colonizing bacteria adhere directly to receptors in the acquired salivary pellicle (Chapter 4). These bacteria compete for binding sites, so a tenaciously adhering bacterial species might effectively exclude other less-adherent species. Therefore, inter-microbial adherence (co-adhesion or co-aggregation) is important because it allows those bacteria that are less competitive in binding to salivary pellicle to nevertheless become incorporated into the biofilm (Figure 14.2). Streptococci and *Actinomyces* are the exemplars of this, frequently binding to each other as well as to salivary pellicle. Co-adherence is mediated by the type 2 fimbriae of *Actinomyces* binding to receptor polysaccharide on the streptococci. As the complex microbial community develops, so components from saliva continue to get incorporated into the matrix. One of the reasons that primary colonizers are often found at different levels throughout plaque is because they bind to salivary components that get deposited onto bacterial cells during the accumulation processes. Bacterial polysaccharides are also important in maintaining the cohesion of plaque.

Co-adhesion

Co-adhesion or co-aggregation is displayed by almost all successful colonizers of plaque that have been tested. Secondary colonizers such as *Fusobacterium* and *P. gingivalis* are especially effective in attaching to earlier plaque colonizers. *Fusobacterium* is very commonly isolated from oral microbial communities. *Fusobacterium* cells express a suite of protein adhesins on their surfaces, such as the arginine-specific RadD, and galactose and N-acetylneuraminic acid-specific lectins which are responsible for intergeneric binding. Multiple direct contacts between bacterial cells lead to a comprehensive network of physical associations being built up. *P. gingivalis* also co-adheres with earlier colonizers such as streptococci and actinomyces, as well as with later colonizers such as

Tannerella forsythia and *Treponema denticola*. Specific adhesion to *S. gordonii* is mediated by two sets of adhesin receptor pairs. The long fimbriae (FimA) bind to glyceraldehyde-3-phosphate dehydrogenase present on the streptococcal surface, and the short fimbriae (Mfa) engage the streptococcal SspA and SspB (Antigen I/II) adhesins. Finding new compounds to disrupt co-aggregation might enable control of the development of microbial communities (Figure 14.3).

Metabolic associations

Oral bacteria tend to accumulate into communities that are metabolically compatible. This can be manifest as simple protection whereby facultative anaerobes such as streptococci remove oxygen that is toxic for the anaerobic secondary colonizing periodontal organisms. Nutritional interrelationships among oral bacteria are common. One of the best defined is between *Veillonella* and *Streptococcus*. Lactate produced by streptococci is utilized directly by *Veillonella* for growth. *Veillonella* lack a fully functional glycolytic pathway; therefore hydroxyl acids e.g. lactate, or carboxylic acids e.g. malate, provide sources of carbon and energy. Thus, levels of *Veillonella* in plaque usually increase with numbers of streptococci. Moreover, as lactate is removed from the immediate environment by *Veillonella*, so the flux of glucose to lactate increases, thus enhancing growth of streptococci. Such co-dependent nutritional associations may account, at least in part, for the difficulty in cultivating a large percentage of the oral microbes.

Antagonism

Not all interbacterial interactions are conducive to mutual colonization. Competition for nutrients and for attachment sites are examples of interbacterial antagonistic relationships. Many oral streptococci produce hydrogen peroxide that can damage and kill other bacteria through the generation of oxidizing free radicals. Streptococci and a variety of oral bacteria including *A. actinomycetemcomitans* produce bacteriocins that are lethal to other bacteria. Actinobacillin, produced by *A. actinomycetemcomitans* is toxic to streptococci and actinomyces and may contribute to the inverse relationship between levels of *A. actinomycetemcomitans* and streptococci/actinomyces in the plaque of patients with localized aggressive periodontitis. Lantibiotics are a class of bacteriocins that contain the post-translationally modified amino acids lanthionine and/or methyllanthionine, and are produced by various members of the oral streptococci. For example, Salivaricin A is produced by *S. salivarius* and is toxic to most strains of *S. pyogenes*. Contact-dependent signaling is also involved in antagonistic interactions. Initial contact between *P. gingivalis* and arginine deiminase on the surface of *Streptococcus cristatus* results in activation of a regulatory cascade that decreases transcription of the gene for FimA. As a result, biofilm accretion does not occur with *P. gingivalis* and *S. cristatus*.

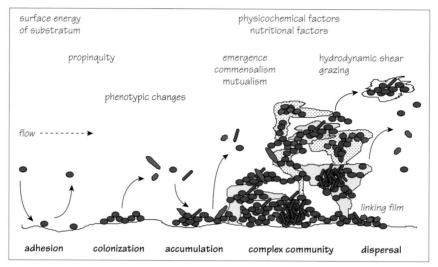

Figure 15.1 Process of biofilm formation. Reproduced with permission from Jenkinson HF, Lappin-Scott HK Biofilms adhere to stay. *Trends in Microbiology* (2001): 9, 9–10.

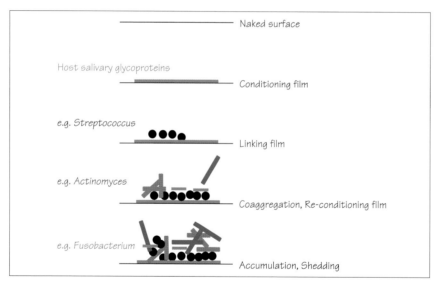

Figure 15.2 Stages in the formation of an oral biofilm community.

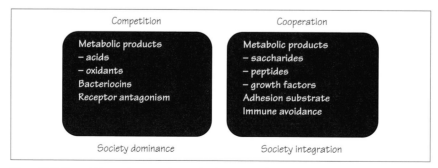

Figure 15.3 Competition and cooperation mechanisms in a multi-society community.

Bacteria in their natural environments do not generally exist as isolated cells, but grow and survive in organized communities. The microbial communities that develop at phase interfaces, such as solid/liquid or air/liquid, are termed biofilms. One feature of biofilms is that microbial cells with very different metabolic requirements can exist successfully in communities. The collective strength of a microbial biofilm community in terms of metabolic efficiency and survival is much greater than the sum of the components. In this respect, the biofilm could be considered as an evolutionary unit.

Biofilm development

The life of an oral biofilm may be depicted as a developmental cycle (Figure 15.1). The various stages of the cycle are determined by physical, biological and environmental factors. Initial adhesion of microbial cells to a biologically conditioned surface, e.g. saliva coated tooth enamel, is a random event influenced by surface free energy and propinquity (nearness) of bacterial cells. If microbial cells adhere, then phenotypic changes occur as the cells divide and form accumulations, generating a linking film. Onto this linking film, new microbial cells may attach and further accumulations of cells occur. During the development of polymicrobial populations, such as dental plaque, every new organism that binds to the linking film presents a new surface (Figure 15.2). This therefore forms the basis for accretion of defined organism groupings. The linking film also provides a means for stabilizing microbial communities that are continuously subject to physical shear forces, e.g. fluid flow, tongue movement. The biofilm community is a dynamic entity: cells continually enter or leave the community, promoting diversification or dispersal, while protozoal grazing and shear forces in flow systems, such as in the oral cavity, lead to biofilm structure remodeling. Within biofilms, constituent species can be in competition or can co-operate with one another (Figure 15.3). Constraints on biofilm accumulation may be beneficial by maintaining an optimal surface area/volume ratio to facilitate diffusion of nutrients and removal of metabolic end-products.

Microbial recognition of surfaces and interbacterial communication

The metabolic processes occurring within microbes undergoing growth on a surface are vastly different from those occurring within microbes in liquid suspension (planktonic). Surface growth is associated with global changes in gene expression. Between 30–50% of genes transcribed in bacteria or fungi can be affected following attachment to substrata. Changes in gene expression result from sensing and recognition of abiotic surfaces and other bacteria, and through interbacterial communication systems. In biofilms, microbial cells in close proximity send signals to each other, such as acyl homoserine lactones (AHLs) in Gram-negative bacteria (although generally not oral Gram-negatives), oligopeptides in Gram-positive bacteria (e.g. CSP, see Chapter 18), or AI-2 (produced by the action of the LuxS enzyme) in both Gram-positives and Gram-negatives. These signaling molecules can act as cell-density-dependent regulators of gene expression and metabolism. They play roles in extracellular polysaccharide (EPS) matrix deposition, maintenance of optimal biofilm architecture and dispersal of bacteria from biofilms. For example, AI-2 dependent polysaccharide synthesis by *S. gordonii* is necessary for optimal heterotypic biofilm formation with *P. gingivalis*. In addition, contact between the Mfa fimbriae of *P. gingivalis* and the AgI/II family protein (SspA/B) of *S. gordonii* initiates a phosphorylation dependent signal transduction cascade in *P. gingivalis* that regulates EPS production and AI-2 levels. *Veillonella atypica* communicates with *S. gordonii* by means of a short-range diffusible signal that increases amylase production in *S. gordonii*, thus providing additional fermentation substrates for *V. atypica*.

The biofilm matrix, resilience and resistance

Many biofilms contain extracellular polymeric materials that contribute to structural integrity. A major component of the *Aggregatibacter actinomycetemcomitans* biofilm matrix is poly-β-1, 6-N-acetyl-D-glucosamine (PGA), a hexosamine-containing polysaccharide that mediates intercellular adhesion. Extracellular DNA also contributes to the matrix in *A. actinomycetemcomitans* biofilms. The role of glucans in *S. mutans* biofilms is discussed in Chapter 16.

The increased resistance properties of biofilm cells to external influences such as antibiotics, host defenses, antiseptics and shear forces, are of major concern in dentistry, medicine and industry. Extracellular polymeric substances, while providing mechanical strength, do not necessarily provide a barrier to inhibitory compounds. Bacteria within biofilms can be inherently more resistant to antimicrobial compounds. For example, small colony variants of *Staphylococcus aureus*, generated within biofilm communities on medical devices, have diminished metabolic rates that make them less susceptible to antibiotics. It is probable that these so-called persister cells with reduced antibiotic susceptibility are commonly produced within biofilms. In mixed biofilms, one β-lactamase producing bacterial species may protect cells of another species from penicillin, while streptococci or staphylococci growing in mixed biofilms with *Candida albicans*, reduce the susceptibility of *C. albicans* to antifungal agents. One of the many challenges is to devise effective means to prevent biofilm infections of indwelling medical devices. Impregnation of biomaterials with slow-release antimicrobials is one approach.

16 Bacterial polysaccharides

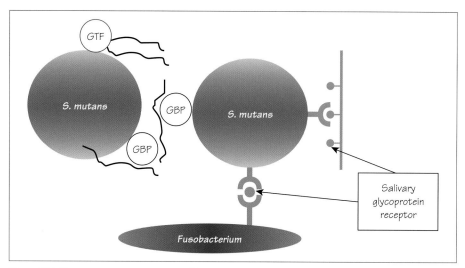

Figure 16.1 Diagrammatic representation of bacterial polysaccharides, synthesized by GTF enzymes, facilitating build up of communities through recognition by glucan binding proteins (GBP). Salivary glycoprotein receptor provides a substrate for adherence to tooth surfaces and for co-adhesion with other bacteria.

Glucans – chains of glucose residues

Linear	Glu-Glu-Glu-Glu-
Branched (less soluble)	Glu-Glu-Glu-Glu- | Glu-Glu-

Fructans – chains of fructose residues

Figure 16.2 Polysaccharides produced by S. mutans from sucrose.

Table 16.1 Properties of glucans produced by S. mutans.

Streptococcus mutans produces from sucrose

(1) Water-soluble glucans

    (a) Readily degraded for energy source

    (b) Formation of lactic acid

(2) Water-insoluble glucans

    (a) Sticky and hard, act as cement

    (b) Promote accumulation of plaque

Many of the oral bacteria produce polysaccharides. Streptococcus strains produce extracellular polysaccharides (EPS) which are usually glucose or fructose polymers. They also accumulate intracellular polysaccharides that are glucose polymers, rather similar in structure to liver glycogen. Actinomyces strains produce mixed sugar polysaccharides. Bacterial polysaccharides provide a matrix that facilitates the accumulation of oral biofilms (Figure 16.1).

Extracellular polysaccharide production

Although EPS production is less important for development of subgingival plaque, it is significant in enhancing colonization of *S. mutans* and other streptococci associated with dental caries (enamel caries and root caries). Bacterial polysaccharides are synthesized by enzymes termed glycosyltransferases. *S. mutans* and several other viridans group streptococci, e.g. *S. salivarius* and *S. gordonii*, can express a number of different enzymes that are active in the synthesis of glucans (chains of glucose residues) and fructans (fructose polymers). The glucan chains may be either linear, or contain branches of chains (Figure 16.2). The branched chains are usually less soluble than the linear chains, and they need more complex sets of enzymes for degradation (Table 16.1). The linear chains are broken down more easily than branched chains by dextranases (DexA in *S. mutans*). The released sugars are taken up by the cells for growth. The glucose sub-units in linear glucan are generally linked by α-1,6 O-glycosidic bonds. α-1,3 bonds cause branched linkages and increased insolubility. α-1,4 linkages are less common as these are a target for digestion by salivary amylase. Fructans can be degraded by fructanase and are a good source of energy for bacteria, as fructose metabolism is quicker and requires one less phosphorylation step than glucose in the glycolytic pathway.

Glycosyltransferases and fructosyltransferases

Glucans and fructans are produced from sucrose (disaccharide of glucose and fructose). Water soluble glucans are produced both inside and outside the cells by glucosyltransferase (GTF) enzymes. These provide a mechanism for the bacteria to conserve sucrose, when it is in good supply (e.g. after meals or sugary drinks), by converting excess sucrose into glucans. Glucans can be broken down later into glucose residues a few hours after dietary intake has ceased. Water insoluble glucans are produced outside the cells. These are more long-term storage compounds, more difficult to break down, but therefore longer lasting in the oral environment. These glucans are sticky and so they can cement plaque together and promote development of microbial communities within a matrix of polysaccharides. GTF enzymes are produced by streptococci and are secreted onto the bacterial cell surface as well as into the environment and can remain active on tooth surfaces. The mechanism of action is first cleavage of sucrose into glucose and fructose. Then, in a two-step reaction, the glucose is added onto the end of a growing polysaccharide chain using the energy released from cleavage of the disaccharide bond. Some enzymes specifically synthesize linear chains (e.g. GtfC and GtfD of *S. mutans*), others catalyze production of a mixture of linear and branched chains (e.g. GtfB of *S. mutans*). The enzymes all have an amino acid repeat block structure running through the carboxy terminal half of the protein. These repeats, designated YG repeats (Y, tyrosine; G, glycine), form the glucan binding domain while enzyme activity is in the amino terminus region. Fructosyltransferases (FTF) specifically make fructan chains and these are often linear (β-2,1 and β-2,6 linkages).

Glucan binding proteins

GTF enzymes on their own are useful for making polysaccharide, but for the polysaccharide to be effective as a storage source of energy it has to be held onto by the cells. To do this the bacteria express glucan-binding proteins (GBPs). These are essentially lectins that bind glucans. GBPs are found on the cell surface of *S. mutans*, and some other streptococci. Some GBPs contain sequences that are similar to the YG repeats in GTFs. In addition to holding onto the polysaccharide for the bacteria to digest, they act as additional cementing agents in the build up of plaque. The GBPs are necessary for optimal *S. mutans* biofilm formation and antibodies raised to GBPs can be protective against development of caries by *S. mutans* in animal studies.

EPS produced by oral Gram-negatives

EPS can be produced by Gram-negative anaerobes such as *P. gingivalis*. At least six polysaccharide capsular serotypes are produced by *P. gingivalis*. The EPS capsule protects against phagocytosis and tends to be lost on laboratory subculture. Antibodies to *P. gingivalis* EPS are protective in animal models. EPS is also involved in *P. gingivalis*-*S. gordonii* biofilm development. *P. gingivalis* EPS can mask LPS and reduce its activity.

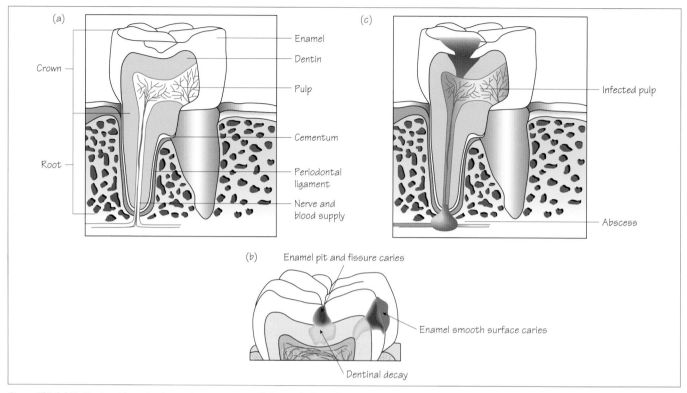

Figure 17.1 (a) Vertical sections showing major components of the tooth. Caries begins as reversible demineraliztion (white spot). (b) If demineralization continues, the enamel decays and destruction eventually spreads through the dentin to the pulp chamber, which can lead to a periapical abscess (c).

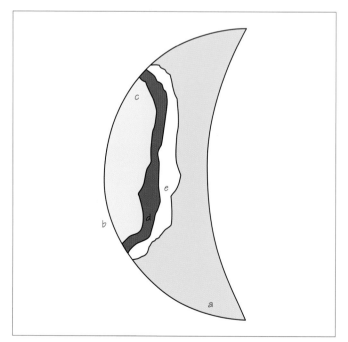

Figure 17.2 Schematic of a section through an early caries lesion on a smooth enamel surface. (a) Sound enamel. (b) Surface enamel slightly demineralized, but appears intact. (c) Body of the lesion with loss of about 25% mineral. (d) Dark zone with loss of about 5% of mineral. (e) Translucent zone with about 1% enamel loss.

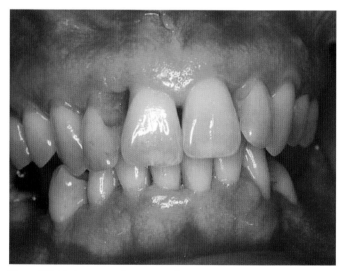

Figure 17.3 Early stages of root caries (discoloration) presenting on multiple teeth.

Dental caries is under control in many human populations. However, there are still major problems with dental decay in children regularly fed high sugar diets or drinks. There are also small populations throughout the world where good dental hygiene is not practiced. A change in diet towards higher sugar intake in these instances is very conducive to caries onset.

Structure of teeth (Figure 17.1)

The surface layer of the coronal part (crown) of the tooth is composed of enamel, a substituted hydroxyapatite (crystalline calcium phosphate). Enamel is highly mineralized and is the hardest substance in the body. Supporting the enamel is dentin, a less mineralized organic matrix of collagenous proteins. Beneath the dentin is the pulp chamber that contains blood vessels and nerves and extends down into the gum as root canals. The roots are composed of dentin and covered with cementum which is a hydroxyapatite and collagen matrix, and is about half as mineralized as enamel. Dentin has microscopic channels, called dentinal tubules, which radiate outward from the pulp chamber to the exterior cementum or enamel border.

Dental caries

Dental caries is the localized destruction of the tissues of the tooth by bacterial action (Figure 17.1). Enamel or cementum is demineralized by microbial acids (predominantly lactic acid) produced by fermentation of dietary sugars. The initial caries lesion is sub-surface, due to acid diffusion (Figure 17.2). The primary lesion that is detectable clinically is known as a white spot and can be reversed by remineralization and regrowth of hydroxyapatite crystals, a process enhanced by fluoride. Advanced caries results in cavitation, and can progress to the dentin and into the pulp chamber ultimately causing necrosis and periapical abscesses.

Types of dental caries

The differing topology and degree of mineralization of the different tissues of the tooth provide unique challenges to bacteria with cariogenic potential.

(1) **Enamel smooth surface caries** These surfaces are easy to keep clean and are continuously exposed to saliva, and thus difficult for bacteria to colonize.

(2) **Pit and fissure and interproximal caries** Bacteria can become physically entrapped in these areas without specialized adherence mechanisms.

(3) **Root caries** Cementum (or dentin when cementum is lost) is more easily demineralized than enamel (Figure 17.3). Roots become exposed to oral bacteria as the gingiva recedes with age or after periodontal surgery. Root caries is thus becoming more prevalent.

(4) **Recurrent caries** This occurs around existing restorations.

(5) **Rampant caries** This involves widespread and severe lesions, usually in people with reduced salivary flow (xerostomia).

(6) **Early childhood caries (nursing or baby bottle caries)** This is rampant caries of the primary dentition of infants and toddlers. The exact causal mechanisms are uncertain but unrestricted access to night-time bottles with fruit juice or sweetened formula is a major contributor.

Important bacteria in caries

Streptococcus mutans

Gram-positive cocci in chains. More accurately, a collection of closely related species known as mutans streptococci and comprising seven species and eight serotypes, a–h. *S. mutans* serotypes c, e and f and *S. sobrinus* serotypes d and g are most closely associated with human disease. *S. cricetus, S. ferus, S. rattus, S. macacae* and *S. downei* are more usually found in animals. Mutans streptococci possess adhesins for salivary receptors allowing attachment to saliva-coated smooth surfaces. In addition, these organisms produce extracellular polysaccharides from sucrose that facilitate retention on surfaces (these virulence factors are discussed in more detail in Chapters 16 and 18). Mutans streptococci are associated with all forms of caries.

Lactobacilli

Gram-positive rods. lactobacilli are efficient producers of lactic acid and are tolerant to low pH values (two important caries associated traits, Chapter 18). However, lactobacilli are poor colonizers of smooth surfaces and probably do not initiate caries at these sites. Most likely lactobacilli are secondary colonizers of established caries lesions, where their aciduric properties allow them to out compete other organisms. Acid production will then exacerbate the lesion and facilitate extension into the dentin. If lactobacilli become embedded in pits and fissures they may be able to initiate caries at these sites. Different species and strains of lactobacilli exhibit differing cariogenic potential.

Actinomyces species

Gram-positive rods. Actinomyces, especially *A. naeslundii*, are frequently isolated from root caries lesions and can cause root caries in experimental animals. However, the organisms are also commonly found on healthy root surfaces so the role of actinomyces in the disease process has been unclear. More recent molecular detection techniques (see below) are re-establishing the importance of *Actinomyces* species in both root and coronal caries.

Emerging and polymicrobial pathogens

Culture independent molecular based techniques such as 16S rRNA sequencing are altering our view of caries etiology. Bacteria that are emerging as important in caries progression include species of the genera *Veillonella, Bifidobacterium,* and *Propionibacterium* and *Atopobium,* along with low-pH non-mutans streptococci. Putative etiological agents of root caries are now thought to include species of *Atopobium, Olsenella, Pseudoramibacter, Propionibacterium* and *Selenomonas.* Dentinal caries is associated with *Rothia dentocariosa* and *Propionibacterium* spp. The collective outcome of these studies is shifting our understanding of caries toward a complex community disease.

18 Virulence factors of *S. mutans*

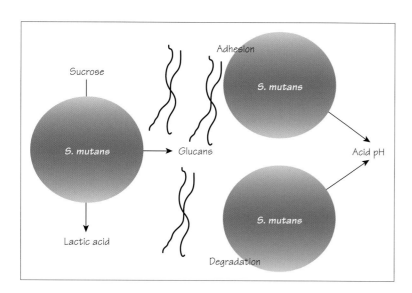

Figure 18.1 *The combined effects of sucrose utilization, glucan production, adhesion and production of lactic acid in the generation of dental caries.*

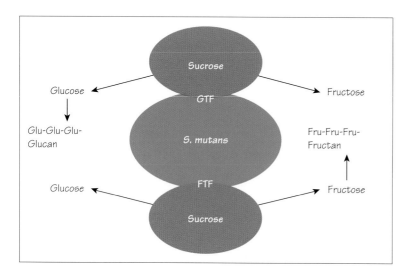

Figure 18.2 *Glucosyltransferase (GTF) and fructosyltransferase (FTF) on the surface of S. mutans synthesize glucans and fructans from sucrose with the release of fructose (GTF) or glucose (FTF).*

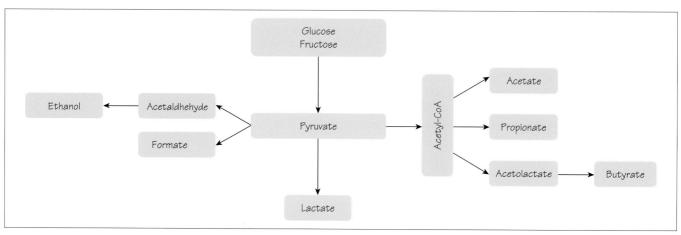

Figure 18.3 *Simplified pathway showing major end products derived from hexose sugars via pyruvate in glycolytic fermentation. Streptococci such as S. mutans are usually homofermentative in producing lactate from glucose or fructose. Fructose fermentation is more efficient than that of glucose.*

S. mutans possess several attributes that contribute to its success as a cariogenic organism: (1) ability to adhere to the tooth surface and develop plaque communities; (2) production of glucans and other polysaccharides from excess carbohydrate (often sucrose) in the diet, leading to plaque accumulation; (3) production of acids (principally lactic acid), that generate a low pH environment and enrich for aciduric organisms (Figure 18.1). Organisms such as *Lactobacilli* that produce and tolerate large amounts of lactic acid are not thought to be the initiators of smooth surface caries as they lack specialized colonization mechanisms. Actinomyces and non-mutans streptococci produce less acid and so may be more important in root caries as cementum (and dentin) is less mineralized and thus more easily dissolved, as compared to enamel.

Initial attachment to tooth surfaces

A major surface protein produced by *S. mutans* is the AgI/II family protein called SpaP (or P1). This protein contributes to the fibrillar layer that is on the outside of *S. mutans* cells, made up of proteins, polysaccharides and teichoic acids. The AgI/II polypeptide of *S. mutans* mediates attachment to salivary pellicle, principally through binding to gp340. AgI/II contains approximately 1500 amino acid residues, and several different regions that bind to salivary glycoproteins, collagen and fibronectin. *S. mutans* can also adhere to earlier colonizing streptococci, a process that can be enhanced by bridging gp340 molecules.

Polysaccharide production

As discussed in Chapter 16, *S. mutans* produces polymers of glucan and fructan from dietary sucrose through glucosyl- and fructosyl-transferases (Figure 18.2). *S. mutans* produces three glucosyltransferases designated GtfB, GtfC and GtfD, and one fructosyltransferase (Ftf). Glucan and fructan can serve as reserves of fermentable carbohydrate, allowing *S. mutans* to continue to metabolize and produce acid when dietary carbohydrates are no longer available. *S. mutans* possesses four glucan binding proteins (Chapter 16), GbpA, B, C and D, and so insoluble glucan also contributes to the cohesiveness and retention of *S. mutans*-rich plaque. Within the cytoplasm, glucose can be polymerized into intracellular polysaccharide (IPS), a glycogen-like polymer that can be mobilized for glycolysis and extend the duration of acidification.

Acid production

S. mutans can metabolize a variety of sugars, resulting in the production of a number of weak acids, including lactic, formic and acetic acids (Figure 18.3). Lactic acid is the strongest of these acids, with an ionization constant (pK_a) of 3.5. When the plaque pH drops below about 5.5 the balance between enamel demineralization and remineralization shifts toward solubility and the caries process is initiated. Sucrose is the most cariogenic sugar because it can be processed into glucan and fructan, and because it is efficiently fermented into lactic acid. Sucrose and other sugars are transported into *S. mutans* cells by the high affinity and high capacity phosphenolpyruvate (PEP) sugar: phosphotransferase (PTS) uptake system. Sucrose is accumulated as sucrose-6-phosphate which is then hydrolyzed to glucose-6-phosphate and fructose which are metabolized via the glycolytic pathway. *S. mutans* also has other sugar uptake systems including proton motive force (PMF) driven transport. Glycolysis of one C6 sugar yields two molecules of pyruvate (C3). The enzyme lactate dehydrogenase then converts pyruvate into lactic acid using NADH as an electron donor. Organisms such as *S. mutans* are considered homofermenters in that as much as 90% of pyruvic acid is converted to lactic acid.

Acid tolerance

S. mutans is highly aciduric, and resistance to the adverse effects of low pH is accomplished by several mechanisms: (1) extrusion of H^+ ions from the cell through a proton translocating F_1-F_0 ATPase (this maintains the cytoplasm at a pH closer to physiological levels); (2) increase in the proportion of mono-unsaturated membrane fatty acids, which will decrease proton permeability; (3) conversion of the arginine derivative agmatine to putrescine, ammonia and CO_2 by the agmatine deiminase system (AgDS); (4) malolactic fermentation, whereby the dicarboxylic L-malate, a major acid in fruits, is converted to the monocarboxylic lactic acid and CO_2; (5) up-regulation of molecular chaperones, proteases and DNA repair enzymes.

Biofilm adaptation

S. mutans is adapted to the biofilm lifestyle and there is coordinated production of bacteriocins along with an increase in competence in high density situations. *S. mutans* may thus acquire DNA from other organisms in close proximity either for nutrition or increasing genetic diversity or both. These processes are controlled by competence stimulating peptide (CSP), a 21-amino-acid peptide pheromone. CSP is a quorum sensing (QS) signal that is secreted into the milieu and initiates transcriptional activity in the bacterial cells after exceeding a threshold level. Biofilm formation and metabolic activity are controlled on multiple levels. Many environmental signals funnel through the nutritional alarmone (p)ppGpp. There are also multiple two-component signal transduction systems (TCS) in the organism, such as the ComDE TCS that responds to CSP.

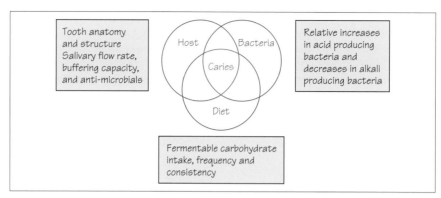

Figure 19.1 Interdependence and requirement for cariogenic bacteria, provided with a fermentable substrate in a susceptible host in order for caries to occur.

Table 19.1 Measurable parameters that are associated with risk of caries development.

Low caries risk	High caries risk
Alkali producing bacteria such as S. sanguinis	Acid producing bacteria such as mutans streptococci and lactobacilli
Unstimulated salivary flow rate > 1 ml/min	Unstimulated salivary flow rate < 0.7 ml/min
Infrequent sucrose consumption	Frequent consumption of high levels of sucrose and other fermentable carbohydrates particularly in retentive forms
Fluoride intake to levels allowing production of fluorapatite	Little or no fluoride intake

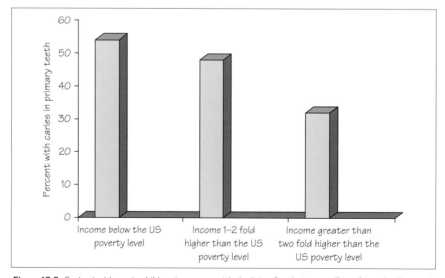

Figure 19.2 Caries incidence in children increases with declining family income. Data from the National Health and Nutrition Examination Survey (NHANES, 1999–2004).

The initiation and progression of caries requires that host, diet and bacterial factors are all conducive to disease (Figure 19.1). In this chapter, host and dietary factors will be considered.

Host factors

(1) Teeth Teeth become less susceptible to caries over time. Such post-eruptive resistance is due in part to an increase in the concentration of fluoride in the surface layer of enamel. Fluoride ions substitute for hydroxyl ions in hydroxyapatite, forming fluorapatite which is less soluble in acid than hydroxyapatite (Chapter 20). Tooth morphology also contributes to caries susceptibility on the basis of ease of bacteria colonization and accessibility to saliva as discussed in Chapter 17.

(2) Saliva There are several important aspects of saliva that contribute to caries resistance:

(a) Flow rate The flow of saliva physically washes away weakly attached bacteria and acids, and delivers salivary buffers. Xerostomia (low salivary flow, < 0.1 ml/min) leads to rampant caries. Xerostomia can be the result of Sjögren's syndrome, or occur after radiation for head and neck cancer when the salivary glands are damaged. Methamphetamine use also damages salivary glands and methamphetamine users often experience severe oral health problems. Certain medications can reduce salivary flow, particularly psychoactive drugs.

(b) Buffering capacity Saliva has two major buffering systems: bicarbonate-carbonic acid and phosphate. Bicarbonate is the most important as it buffers rapidly and is effective at pH values found in plaque. Buffering by saliva helps prevent bacterial acids, from reducing the pH to levels that dissolve apatite. The levels of ammonia and urea in saliva may also contribute to resistance to pH decline.

(c) Supersaturation At physiological pH saliva is supersaturated with respect to calcium and phosphate. This helps prevent loss of calcium and phosphate from enamel mineral. Anionic proline-rich proteins and a basic proline-rich glycoprotein are responsible for most of the calcium binding. Statherin is an active inhibitor of calcium phosphate precipitation.

(d) Antimicrobial factors Lysozyme, salivary peroxidase, mucins, agglutinins and immunoglobulins (IgA from saliva, IgG and IgM from serum via GCF) all possess antimicrobial properties as discussed in Chapters 6 and 7.

Dietary factors

In order to produce acid, cariogenic bacteria require a fermentable carbohydrate substrate, in particular sucrose. Studies have shown that in addition to total consumption, the frequency of intake and physical form of the sucrose containing food are important. The classical Vipeholm study found that in an institutionalized population the retentiveness of the food and frequency of intake were more important than total sucrose consumption.

The potential cariogenicity of food can be assessed by measuring the pH changes in plaque over time following ingestion. In general, there is a rapid pH drop followed by a slow rise back to resting pH, a pattern known as the Stephan curve after the first person to perform these measurements. Sucrose, glucose and fructose produce a more sustained and lower pH drop than some other sugars, such as lactose and starch. The bacterial metabolic pathways that lead to acid production from sugars are discussed in Chapter 18. Sucrose has the additional cariogenic property of providing a substrate for bacterial glucosyltransferases and fructosyltransferases. As discussed in Chapter 16, these enzymes produce polymers of glucan and fructan respectively from sucrose, both of which provide long-term energy storage. In addition, glucans can be insoluble and act as a cohesive matrix for the development and retention of cariogenic plaque.

Caries risk assessment

As the etiology of caries has become better understood, attempts have been made to measure known risk factors in order to assess caries risk. This would allow more proactive preventive measures when risk is high, for example in low income populations (Figure 19.2). Also, identification of children at high risk for caries would allow tailored pediatric preventive dentistry. Caries risk assessment should include at a minimum: bacterial factors (*S. mutans* and lactobacilli levels), salivary parameters (flow rate and buffering capacity), and a diet analysis (amount of fermentable carbohydrate). Fluoride levels in saliva and levels of salivary components such as gp340 could also be useful (Table 19.1). Unfortunately there are several drawbacks to these kinds of tests. It is not easy to distinguish the more cariogenic *S. mutans* or lactobacilli strains from less cariogenic strains, although nucleic acid or monoclonal antibody approaches may resolve this issue in the future. Salivary parameters vary considerably according to time of day or emotional state of the patient. An accurate chair-side test is therefore not yet available.

20 Fluoride

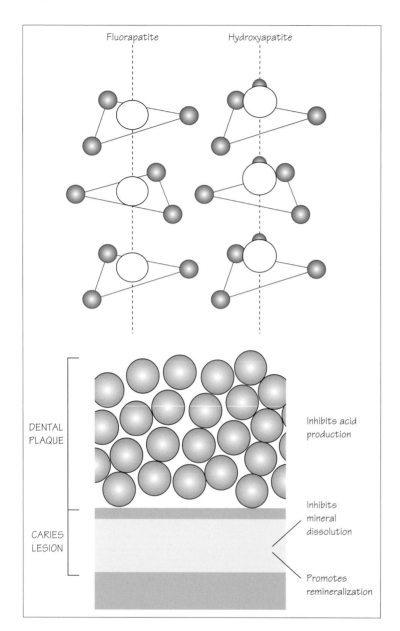

Fluorapatite   Hydroxyapatite

DENTAL PLAQUE

Inhibits acid production

Inhibits mineral dissolution

CARIES LESION

Promotes remineralization

Figure 20.1 Upper panel: Crystal structure showing fluorapatite is a more compact structure than hydroxyapatite. Lower panel: Mechanisms of action of fluoride. Fluoride inhibits acid production and mineral dissolution, and promotes remineralization.

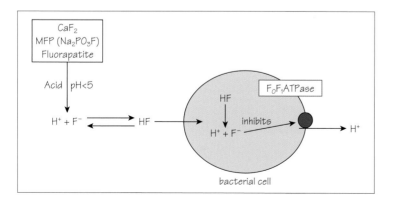

CaF_2
MFP (Na_2PO_3F)
Fluorapatite

Acid | pH<5

$H^+ + F^- \rightleftharpoons HF$

HF

F_0F_1ATPase

HF

$H^+ + F^-$ inhibits

H^+

bacterial cell

Figure 20.2 Fluoride from diet, toothpaste (MFP, sodium monofluorophosphate) or as fluorapatite can be released under low pH (acid). Fluoride ions interact with hydrogen ions to form hydrogen fluoride which enters bacterial cells, Dissociation again into hydrogen and fluoride ions leads to direct inhibition of the major energy and pH regulating transporter protein complex designated F_0F_1ATPase. Inhibition of this leads to the build up of hydrogen ions within the cell and therefore lessens the ability of the cells to tolerate acid (hydrogen ions) in the environment. One mechanism by which fluoride inhibits streptococci is therefore through reducing the ability of the bacterial cells to withstand acidic pH.

All hard tissues (bone, dentin, cementum and enamel) are made up of crystals of mineral (calcium phosphate) together with organic matrix and water. Mineralization of hard tissues is a biologically controled precipitation process. In precipitation, dissolved mineral ions leave a supersaturated solution and aggregate to form solid mineral. The mineral of bones and teeth are impure (partial carbonate substitution for phosphate) forms of hydroxyapatite. This is the least soluble simple calcium phosphate at neutral pH. The structure consists of phosphate (PO_4 $_{3-}$) ions held together by Ca^{2+} ions. The Ca^{2+} ions form triangles and a spiral enclosing a channel. The OH- ions are located inside this channel (see Figure 20.1). In hydroxyapatite, the OH- ions lie slightly outside of the triangles because they are too large to fit exactly. Fluorapatite is formed when F- ions substitute for OH- and is less soluble than hydroxyapatite. In fluorapatite the smaller F- ions fit within the triangles. This results in a more compact and stable structure. Enamel has a much higher mineral content than dentin, resulting in greater density, stiffness and hardness. Because hydroxyapatite and fluorapatite are salts of phosphoric acid, solubility of all these solids increases as pH decreases.

Modes of action of fluoride

The presence of topical fluoride has three major effects (Figure 20.1): (1) Inhibition of acid production by dental plaque (see below). (2) Inhibition of mineral dissolution at the site of carious lesion. Fluoride present in the plaque fluid at the time that the bacteria generate acid will travel with the acid into the subsurface of the tooth and adsorb to the crystal surface protecting against being dissolved. (3) Enhancement of remineralization resulting in a remineralized layer that is less soluble and resistant to acid attack. Fluoride enhances remineralization by adsorbing to the crystal surface and attracting calcium and phosphate ions, leading to new mineral depositing on existing crystal nucleators. This newly formed layer excludes carbonate and is less soluble than carbonated hydroxyapatite.

Strategies for fluoride delivery

Consumption of fluoridated water during tooth development raises the fluoride content of tooth mineral. However, continual local presence of fluoride in the aqueous phase is essential to maintain beneficial effects. Fluoride tablets or clinically-applied topical fluoride boosts the fluoride concentrations of tooth surfaces. Fluoride toothpastes provide reservoirs of fluoride on the tooth surfaces (as calcium fluoride), on mucosa and in plaque (bound to surfaces of bacteria). At dose levels represented by normal dental use, there is no compelling evidence for toxic effects.

Dental fluorosis, caused by impaired mineralization only occurs with very high fluoride concentrations that occur naturally in some water supplies. Mild cases show as white patches of enamel (mottling). In severe cases there is enamel hypomineralization and discoloration due to staining of porous enamel.

Anti-microbial effects of fluoride

Fluoride affects the physiology of microbial cells. There are two main mechanisms: inhibition of enzymes in intact cells, either directly or in the form of metal complexes at sub-millimolar levels; or increasing proton permeability of cell membranes by HF acting as a transmembrane proton carrier, which discharges the ΔpH across the cell membrane (Figure 20.2). This latter effect is the major activity leading to inhibition of acid production by bacterial cells in biofilms at low pH. Lowering of ΔpH by fluoride affects the energy status of the cell. The re-entry of protons across the membrane increases the ATP demand for pH regulation, so the result is intracellular stress.

In addition, fluoride in combination with aluminum inhibits the activity of proton translocating F-ATPase. Cytoplasmic acidification caused by fluoride disrupts glycolytic acid production, and the formation of intracellular storage polysaccharides. Fluoride at low concentrations can also affect the formation of S. mutans biofilms. Reduced extracellular glucan polysaccharide production in these biofilms may be related to partial inhibition of GTF by fluoride. At sub-millimolar levels, fluoride inhibits a variety of enzymes including enolase, urease, P-ATPase, phosphatases and heme peroxidase, by direct binding of HF or F-. Binding of metal-F complexes inhibits F-ATPase and RecA (needed for DNA repair). Dissipation of the proton gradient (as described above) inhibits glycolysis, sugar uptake through the phosphotransferase systems (PTS), and polysaccharide production.

Enhancing anti-microbial effects

The effectiveness of fluoride may be enhanced when combined with other cariostatic agents. Most of the agents used to date to enhance fluoride biological activity are based on non-specific antimicrobial agents such as chlorhexidine, triclosan and metal ions/cations. Two naturally occurring compounds, apigenin and tt-farnesol, found in propolis (a resinous beehive product) and fruits, show inhibitory activities against S. mutans. Apigenin inhibits GTF while tt-farnesol disrupts proton permeability of the cell membrane. These compounds enhance the biological effects of fluoride, reducing the amount of glucans in S. mutans biofilms, the biomass and the acidogenicity.

21 Anti-caries strategies

Table 21.1 Microbial stages in the production of carious lesions, the bacterial factors involved and potential strategies for intervention.

Stages	Bacterial factor	Strategy
Adherence	Antigen I/II	Immunization
Survival and Growth	VikRK	TCS inhibitors
	ComCDE	Natural inhibitors
		Targeted antibacterial peptides
Biofilm	Antigen I/II	Immunization
	LuxS	QS inhibitors
		Photodynamic therapy
		Probiotics
Complex plaque	GTF	Immunization
		Inhibitors
Accumulation	GTF	Immunization
	GBP	
Acid	LDH	Probiotics
	DexA	Xylitol
Dental caries		Fluoride

Table 21.2 Caries immunization strategies

Immunization*	Host	Effect
Killed whole cells of S. mutans (parenteral) (A)	Monkey	Protection against S. mutans induced caries
Purified surface antigens I/II and WapA (Antigen III) (parenteral) (A)	Rodent Monkey	Protection against S. mutans induced caries
Monoclonal antibody to Antigen I/II (oral) (P)	Monkey Human	Prevents colonization or re-colonization by S. mutans
Hen-egg antibody to killed whole S. mutans cells (digestive tract) (P)	Human	Inhibits colonization by mutans streptococci
IgA Fab antibody to Antigen I/II from transgenic tobacco plants (digestive tract) (P)	Monkey	Inhibits colonization by mutans streptococci
GTF enzymes or fragments (parenteral) (A)	Rodent	Protection against S. mutans induced caries
GBP-B	Rodent	Protection against caries
GBP-B and Antigen I/II peptides in liposomes (nasal spray) (A)	Rodent Human	Protection against caries Proposed trials
Antigen I/II N-terminal fragment coupled to CtxB (cholera toxin B subunit adjuvant) (nasal spray) (A)	Human	Trials

*Active (A) immunization depends upon the application of antigen to generate protective antibodies. Passive (P) immunization is the application of pre-formed antibodies.

Dental caries proceeds through a temporal series of events, sometimes taking many months or years. Caries results from the accumulation of acid-producing dental plaque which develops by bacterial adherence to salivary pellicle, formation of a biofilm containing many species of bacteria, and polysaccharide-mediated accumulation of microorganisms. Plaque removal is effectively practiced by tooth brushing with an abrasive paste. However, inter-proximal plaque is difficult to remove, as is subgingival plaque. The route towards dental caries is shown in Table 21.1. The possible targets (bacterial factors) for control strategies to be applied at each of these stages are also shown.

Inhibitors

Over the years, many studies have been undertaken on the effects of inhibitors at several stages of caries development. There have never been any major attempts to utilize antibiotics to control caries although caries rates are lower in patients on long-term antibiotic therapy, such as tetracycline to control chronic acne. Effective natural inhibitors of microbial growth and biofilm formation include polyphenols (from tea extracts) and catechins (from green tea). High molecular mass components present within cranberry juice inhibit biofilm formation. Apigenin, a naturally occurring flavonoid, is a potent inhibitor of GTFs and reduces *S. mutans* biofilm formation. The precise modes of action of these compounds on oral bacteria are not known. Selectively targeted antimicrobial peptides have been generated by fusion of a species-specific targeting peptide domain (CSP in the case of *S. mutans*) with a wide-spectrum antimicrobial peptide domain (derived from novispirin G10). Xylitol is an artificial sweetener that is taken up by *S. mutans* cells via a fructose transporter and inhibits glycolysis. With the realization that bacteria are able to communicate with each other, and that this is essential for biofilm formation, synthetic inhibitors have been designed that interfere with signal recognition by two-component signal transduction systems (TCS), such as VikKR, or mimic the signaling molecules, thus interfering with QS quorum sensing or LuxS/AI-2 communication. Lastly, photodynamic therapy has been proposed as an effective means to control plaque formation. A chemical photosensitizer, such as toluidine blue, is allowed to become incorporated into biofilms. Bacteria are then killed by irradiation with red light.

Probiotics

Probiotic therapy provides a live microbial supplement that beneficially affects the host's healthy microbial balance. Probiotics have commonly been associated with food supplements, such as *Lactobacillus* and *Bifidobacterium* within yogurts. *Lactobacillus* species have also been shown to have some effect on preventing oral colonization by *S. mutans*. A novel approach to biological control of *S. mutans* has been to engineer a strain that lacks lactate dehydrogenase (does not produce lactic acid) and produces a potent bacteriocin that kills other *S. mutans*. In theory, introduction of this strain into the mouth, will destroy other *S. mutans* but reside harmlessly in plaque unable to produce lactic acid.

Immunization

The generation of antibodies to bacteria, or bacterial virulence factors, has been central to the control of many infections. Immunization may be passive (the application of preformed antibodies) or active (vaccination with antigens to generate antibodies). Passive immunization regimens have been very promising for control of *S. mutans*, but none has yet been brought into practice (Table 21.2). Vaccination of cows or hens with GTF or GBP preparations (see Chapter 16) led to the production of high-titer antibodies to these proteins in milk or eggs. The milk antibodies were found to be very effective at preventing *S. mutans* colonization in animal studies. Antibodies generated in mice to AgI/II were found to be effective in preventing *S. mutans* induced caries in animals. These studies have been extended to producing S-IgA to AgI/II in transgenic plants (plantibodies). The AgI/II antibodies, when applied to professionally cleaned teeth of volunteers, inhibited the re-emergence of *S. mutans* for over a year.

Vaccination

Studies in the 1970s showed that vaccination of laboratory animals with killed cells of *S. mutans* generated antibodies that protected against dental caries. Since then a large body of work has concentrated on developing a potential vaccine for humans. There were many fears of generating autoimmune responses with these whole cell vaccines. Consequently, there has been more emphasis on designing acellular vaccines comprised of surface proteins or antigenic segments of these, or of DNA. Fusion of immunogens to the B sub-unit of cholera toxin as a mucosal adjuvant improves antigen specific memory responses to oral vaccines. Expression of recombinant *S. mutans* antigens in attenuated strains of *Salmonella* is another approach to boost antibody responses. One of the most promising vaccines to date contains small segments of the AgI/II and GbpB linked together. The suggestion is that this might be utilized to vaccinate young children who have been identified as being especially prone to caries. The vaccine could be administered as a nasal spray containing an adjuvant, which stimulates immune cell responses. As such, it has been shown that this generates IgG circulatory antibodies, as well as mucosal IgA antibodies. The idea is that this method of vaccination may induce protection at the oral surface against colonization (through IgA), and provide IgG antibodies that reach the oral cavity following secretion in gingival crevicular fluid.

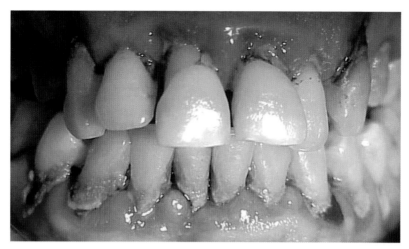

Figure 22.1 *Severe chronic periodontitis with gingival inflammation, bleeding, pus formation and tissue destruction.*

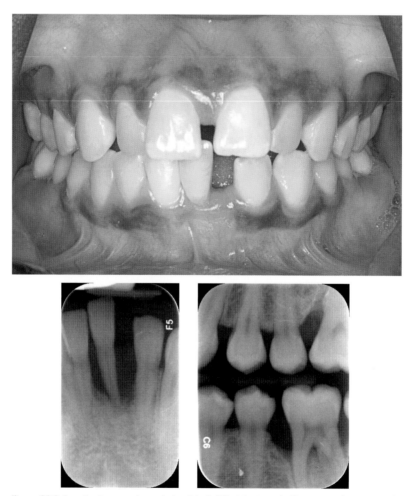

Figure 22.2 *Localized aggressive periodontitis (LAP) with minimal inflammation (upper panel), but bone loss around incisors and first permanent molars is evident on X-ray (lower panels).*

Bacteria in combination with the host inflammatory response are responsible for most forms of periodontal disease. Periodontal diseases are mixed infections and a variety of bacteria or groups of bacteria are required for the initiation and progression of the disease in a susceptible host. The identities of these organisms can vary among diseases, among patients and even among sites in the same patient. These bacteria are often present in healthy individuals, and thus periodontal diseases can be considered opportunistic infections.

The development of periodontal disease is associated with deepening of the gingival crevice into a periodontal pocket that can be several millimeters in depth and bleeds upon probing. Periodontal diseases are very common and it is estimated that over 50% of adults in the USA have experienced some form of the disease, although less than 10% have the severe forms.

Classification of periodontal diseases

There are many different types of periodontal disease. Some of the most common are:

(1) **Gingivitis** Gingivitis is generally the result of overgrowth of supragingival plaque that irritates the gingival tissues. Gingivitis is a reversible inflammation that can be exacerbated by systemic factors, e.g. pregnancy, viral immunosuppression.

(2) **Periodontitis** Periodontitis is an inflammatory-based infection of the supporting structures of the teeth, with progressive destruction of the periodontal ligament and alveolar bone, leading to tooth loss. Periodontitis is the most common cause of adult tooth loss in developed countries. There are two major forms: chronic and aggressive.

   (a) **Chronic periodontitis** This is the most common manifestation, and usually occurs in adults (Figure 22.1). The severity is consistent with local factors of plaque and calculus. It is episodic, with overall slow progression, and can be exacerbated by systemic factors.

   (b) **Aggressive periodontitis** In this case severity is not consistent with local factors of plaque and calculus. There is rapid tissue destruction. A strong genetic component is indicated by the familial pattern of occurrence and differing incidences in ethnic groups (there is a 15-fold higher incidence of LAP in African-American populations as compared to other groups). Aggressive periodontitis can be further subdivided:

      (i) Localized aggressive periodontitis (LAP), formerly known as localized juvenile periodontitis (LJP). The onset of LAP is around puberty, and the disease is restricted to the incisors and first molars. Usually there is little inflammation and individuals may not realize they have the disease until given an X-ray at a later date (Figure 22.2).

      (ii) Generalized aggressive periodontitis (GAP). This manifestation is found in patients under 30, and involves at least three teeth other than incisors and first molars.

(3) **Necrotizing periodontal diseases** These are characterized by painful necrosis of gingival tissues, periodontal ligament and alveolar bone. The disease is often associated with emotional stress (the condition was called "trench mouth" among soldiers in World War I) and with systemic conditions including HIV infection, malnutrition and immunosuppression.

(4) **Peri-implantitis** As the name suggests, this is destruction of tissue and bone surrounding an implant, and similar to chronic periodontitis.

Role of plaque bacteria in periodontal diseases

The metabolic action of early bacterial colonizers in the gingival crevice alters the environment and facilitates colonization by secondary organisms. These secondary colonizers tend to be more pathogenic and when they exceed threshold levels disease can occur. However, the mere presence of periodontopathic bacteria does not necessarily result in disease. The concordance of a variety of bacterial virulence factors, the activity and composition of the commensal microbiota, and host immune factors, are required for the initiation of the disease process (see the Ecological plaque hypothesis in Chapter 9). Periodontal pathogens are discussed in more detail in succeeding chapters.

Role of host factors in periodontal diseases

As with many infections, the pathology associated with periodontal diseases may be caused by immunopathogenic mechanisms. This is discussed further in Chapter 26. Other host factors that can adversely affect periodontal health are: smoking/tobacco use, which disrupts immune function and limits local blood flow; genetics (Chapter 26); pregnancy/puberty, when there are changes in the levels of hormones that can affect the immune response and can be used for nutrition by some pathogenic bacteria; systemic diseases such as diabetes, stress, obesity; and poor nutrition that can affect host immune status. As discussed in Chapter 26, neutrophils are important as a first line of defense against periodontal bacteria, and susceptibility to periodontal disease often correlates with neutrophil deficiencies. Antibodies to periodontal bacteria are also found in serum and in gingival crevicular fluid (GCF) in most forms of the disease, although there is usually a poor antibody response in GAP. The protective function of antibodies in the GCF mainly relates to opsonization and increased phagocytosis. Antibodies to *A. actinomycetemcomitans* (Chapter 23), the predominant pathogen in LAP, may be one reason why the disease is limited to the incisors and first permanent molars. These teeth are the first to erupt into the oral cavity and after infection subsequent antibody production may prevent infection of later erupted teeth and the disease "burns out". Developmental or acquired anatomical deformities can predispose to periodontal disease, particularly those relating to gingival excess that create an environment conducive to the retention of bacteria in the periodontal area.

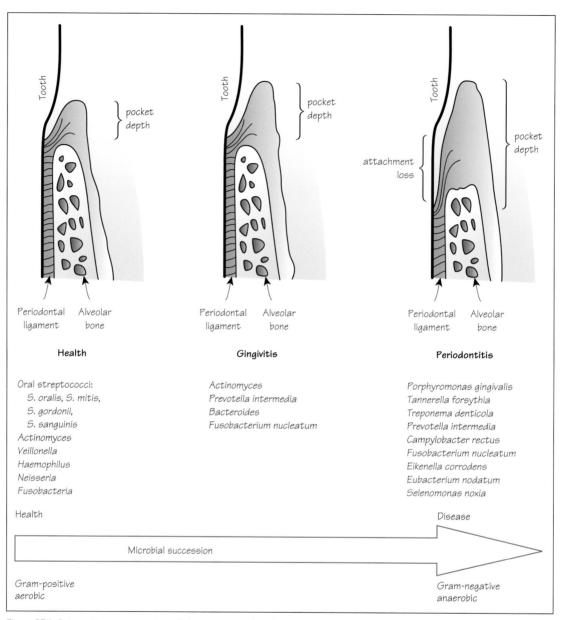

Figure 23.1 Schematic representations of changes in periodontal tissues and bacterial colonizers during disease development. Reproduced in modified form with permission from Lamont RJ, Burne RA, Lantz MS, LeBlanc DJ (eds) *Oral Microbiology and Immunology* (2006) ASM Press, Washington DC.

As discussed in Chapter 22, specific groupings of bacteria are associated with the initiation and progression of different types of periodontal disease (Figure 23.1). The association of these organisms with disease is based on several criteria: elevated numbers in disease compared to health; reduction in numbers following therapy; host responses to the organism in disease; pathogenicity in animal models; and presence of relevant virulence factors. While none of these alone is definitive, the concordance of a number of such attributes increases the likelihood that the organism is a pathogen. It is also important to remember that most of the putative pathogens are also present in healthy mouths and disease requires a shift in the balance between host and organism that allows the pathogenic bacteria to increase in number and express their virulence factors at susceptible sites (Chapter 25).

Gingivitis

The organisms involved in gingivitis tend to also be commonly found in mature supragingival plaque in healthy individuals.

Actinomyces spp: Gram-positive facultatives that comprise a large proportion of the supragingival and subgingival plaque microbiota.

Prevotella intermedia: a Gram-negative black pigmenting anaerobe.

Bacteroides species: Gram-negative anaerobes.

Fusobacterium nucleatum: a Gram-negative anaerobe present in high numbers in supra- and sub-gingival plaque both in health and disease.

Chronic periodontitis

Organisms associated with chronic periodontitis are secondary, often anaerobic, colonizers of mature subgingival plaque that possess tissue destructive properties.

Porphyromonas gingivalis: a highly proteinaceous, asaccharolytic, Gram-negative black pigmenting anaerobe.

Tannerella forsythia: a Gram-negative anaerobe with an outer S-layer.

Treponema denticola and other medium and large size spirochetes. Spirochetes are corkscrew shaped, generally difficult to culture, and are motile by means of their axial filaments/endoflagella.

Prevotella intermedia: see above.

Campylobacter rectus: Gram-negative, motile, anaerobe.

Fusobacterium nucleatum: see above. Different strains or subspecies may exhibit different virulence.

Eikenella corrodens: a Gram-negative facultative. Colonies form pits on agar, hence the name 'corrodens'.

Eubacterium nodatum: a Gram-positive anaerobe.

Selenomonas noxia: Gram-negative, curved rod. Exhibits tumbling motility and has a tuft of flagella in the concave side.

Peptostreptococci: Gram-positive anaerobic cocci.

Herpes viruses: may work synergistically with bacteria.

Localized aggressive periodontitis

LAP is almost exclusively associated with *Aggregatibacter actinomycetemcomitans*, a Gram-negative capnophile.

Generalized aggressive periodontitis

GAP is associated with a subset of organisms involved in chronic periodontitis: *P. gingivalis*, *Tannerella forsythia*, *P. intermedia*, *P. nigrescens* (closely related to *P. intermedia*) and *Selenomonas*.

Color-coded complexes

In the plaque biofilm, groups of metabolically compatible organisms assemble into complexes that have distinct pathogenic potential. It can be instructive, therefore, to color code these complexes according to their potential danger to the host. The most pathogenic of these groupings is the red complex, comprising *P. gingivalis*, *T. forsythia* and *T. denticola*. The complexes also become spatially and temporally associated in developing subgingival plaque.

P. gingivalis, a consensus pathogen

While there is considerable debate over the relative pathogenic status of many oral organisms, most in the field would agree that *P. gingivalis* is among the most pathogenic. *P. gingivalis* is a Gram-negative anaerobic coccobacillus, closely related to the *Bacteroides*, although the organism is fairly aereotolerant and can even grow under low oxygen conditions. Aerotolerance presumably aids transmission of the organism between individuals and early survival in the oral cavity. *P. gingivalis* is asaccharolytic, meaning that it relies on the catabolism of amino acids for energy production and growth. Degradation of proteins and peptides is thus important for the *P. gingivalis* nutrition, and the organisms express a number of proteolytic enzymes with differing specificities. *P. gingivalis* preferentially acquires iron in the form of heme (a ferrous complex found in hemoglobin and other host proteins). The availability of heme regulates virulence expression by the organism (Chapter 25). Heme derivatives accumulate on the bacterial surface, imparting the black pigmented appearance of colonies on blood agar, and help protect against oxidative stress. Indeed, *P. gingivalis* has multiple systems to protect against oxidative stress, including superoxide dismutase, alkyl hydroperoxide reductase, and rubrerythrin. As *P. gingivalis* strains are frequently present in the mouth, regardless of disease status (although in lower numbers in health), *P. gingivalis* is more accurately an opportunistic pathogen. No one clonal type is associated with disease (reflective of a long-term evolutionary relationship between host and micro-organism), although differences in fimbrial type and capsule expression may alter virulence.

A. actinomycetemcomitans, a pathogen in LAP

LAP is almost exclusively associated with *A. actinomycetemcomitans*, a Gram-negative capnophilic (preferring elevated CO_2) coccobacillus. *A. actinomycetemcomitans* is in the *Pasteurellaceae* family, and a member of the HACEK group of pathogens (together with *Haemophilus*, *Cardiobacterium*, *Eikenella* and *Kingella*). Recent clinical isolates tend to be fimbriated (resulting in colonies with a star shape in the center), but production of fimbriae is lost on laboratory sub-culture. Six serotypes (a–f) of the LPS O-polysaccharide are recognized currently, of which serotype b is more commonly associated with disease.

Culture independent bacterial detection

Recent advances in molecular based identification methods have allowed the detection of large numbers of organisms that cannot as yet be cultivated (Chapter 10), and organisms difficult to isolate such as methanogenic Archaea and sulfate-reducing bacteria. Some of these, e.g. the genera *Megasphaera* and *Desulfobulbus*, and *Filifactor alocis* are more abundant in periodontal lesions; however, the pathogenic status of these organisms remain to be established.

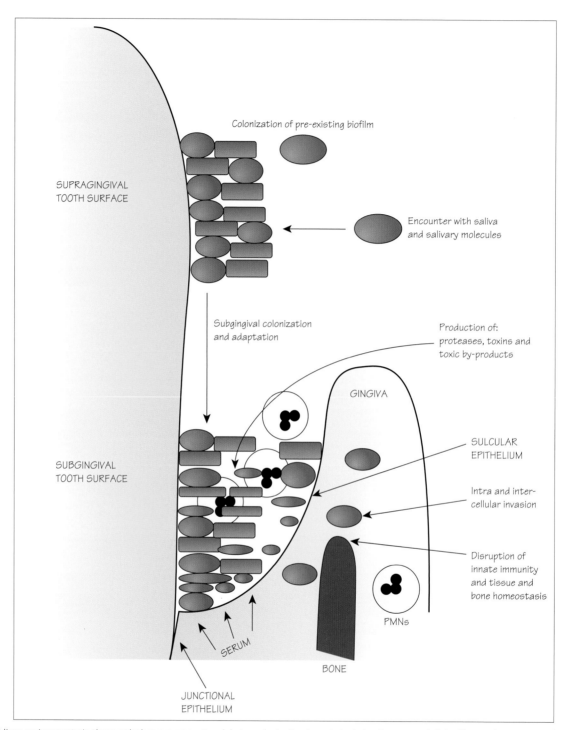

Colonization of pre-existing biofilm

SUPRAGINGIVAL
TOOTH SURFACE

Encounter with saliva
and salivary molecules

Subgingival colonization
and adaptation

Production of:
proteases, toxins and
toxic by-products

GINGIVA

SULCULAR
EPITHELIUM

SUBGINGIVAL
TOOTH SURFACE

Intra and inter-
cellular invasion

Disruption of
innate immunity
and tissue and
bone homeostasis

PMNs

SERUM

BONE

JUNCTIONAL
EPITHELIUM

Figure 24.1 Micro-environments in the mouth that are encountered during colonization by periodontal pathogens and their effect on host tissues. Reproduced with permission from Lamont RJ, Burne RA, Lantz MS, LeBlanc DJ (eds) *Oral Microbiology and Immunology* (2006) ASM Press, Washington DC.

Oral bacteria are acquired shortly after birth, usually from a care giver, and transmission through close contact continues throughout life. Motile organisms such as spirochetes can be chemotactically attracted to compounds in the gingival crevice. Non-motile organisms adhere to available surfaces and then reach the subgingival crevice by spreading proliferation from the supragingival surfaces or translocation of dislodged progeny if at a remote site (Figure 24.1).

Adhesion

Periodontal pathogens tend to be later colonizers and adhere to antecedent colonizers and their products. Periodontal bacteria also adhere to the oral soft tissues, either to the epithelial cells directly or to the extracellular matrix.

Periodontal bacterial adhesins

P. gingivalis possesses two (at least) distinct fimbriae. The long fimbriae are comprised of the FimA structural protein and mediate attachment to salivary proline-rich proteins and statherin; early colonizers such as *S. gordonii*; epithelial cells, endothelial cells and fibroblasts; and matrix proteins such as fibronectin and fibrinogen. Many of these binding properties have been located to discrete linear domains in the FimA sub-unit. The long fimbriae are classified into six genotypes (I to V and Ib) on the basis of the diversity of the *fimA* genes. The shorter fimbriae are comprised of the Mfa protein and mediate attachment to other bacteria. *P. gingivalis* expresses two proteins of the Internalin J class of leucine rich repeat (LRR) proteins that are involved in adhesion and biofilm formation. *P. gingivalis* also produces a series of hemagglutinins that bind to host cells, and proteinases (Chapter 25) that possess hemagglutinin domains that can also be involved in adhesion.

A. actinomycetemcomitans possesses the type IV Flp fimbriae that are responsible for non-specific adherence and biofilm formation on solid surfaces, including saliva coated surfaces. The Flp fimbriae are assembled and secreted through the activities of *tad* gene products, a locus that is widespread in other bacteria and archaea. The *tad* locus is on a genomic island and contains 14 genes necessary for the biogenesis of the fimbriae. The Flp fimbriae are readily lost on laboratory subculture and the colonies change from a rough to a smooth appearance. Specific adhesion of *A. actinomycetemcomitans* to epithelial cells is mediated by the autotransporter proteins Aae and ApiA. The extracellular matrix protein adhesin A (EmaA), also an autotransporter, mediates binding to collagen.

An important adhesin of *T. denticola* is a major outer membrane protein Msp, which mediates attachment to matrix proteins and cells. Msp is also a porin and can become integrated into the membranes of host cells with resultant cytotoxicity. In conjunction with proteases (discussed below) Msp degrades the integrity of the periodontium and allows *T. denticola* to invade periodontal tissues.

The RadD outer membrane protein is responsible for arginine-inhibitable adherence of *F. nucleatum* and contributes to coadhesion with other oral bacteria and multispecies biofilm formation. The leucine rich adhesin FadA is responsible for epithelial cell attachment and entry by *F. nucleatum*. FadA is anchored in the inner membrane and protrudes through the outer membrane.

T. forsythia has yet to be investigated in as much detail as some of the other periodontal pathogens. A major adhesin is BspA, a member of the LRR protein family that mediates adherence to host cells and matrix proteins, and to other bacteria. BspA is also required for *T. forsythia* induced bone loss in animals and for entry into epithelial cells.

Intracellular invasion

Adhesion to host cells can be a prelude to internalization. In non-professional phagocytes such as epithelial cells this is a bacterially driven process. Epithelial cells recovered from the oral cavity can contain large numbers of bacteria, indicating that this is an important *in vivo* process.

Mechanisms of invasion

Invasion of *P. gingivalis* is initiated by the interaction of the FimA fimbriae with integrin receptors on gingival epithelial cells. Integrin-dependent signaling, along with signaling induced by a secreted *P. gingivalis* serine phosphatase (SerB), results in remodeling of the host microfilament and microtubule cytoskeleton that is necessary for bacterial engulfment through lipid raft components. Subversion of host cell signal transduction through phosphorylation/dephosphorylation of proteins and calcium ion fluxes allows trafficking of *P. gingivalis* to the perinuclear area and ultimately impacts gene expression in the host cells. Internalized *P. gingivalis* remain viable and undergo major shifts in physiological status, with around 40% of the expressed proteome differentially regulated as the organism adapts to an intracellular environment. *P. gingivalis* suppresses apoptotic cell death through inhibition of intrinsic (mitochondrial) apoptotic pathways, and accelerates progression of epithelial cells through the cell cycle. *P. gingivalis* can spread to uninfected cells through actin based intercellular protrusions and thus prevent removal from the tissue following host cell death and sloughing.

Host responses to intracellular bacteria

Epithelial cells respond to internalized bacteria through gene expression changes that are tailored to the infecting organism. These can have consequences for innate immunity, e.g. *P. gingivalis* suppresses expression of the neutrophil chemokine Interleukin (IL)-8, which will compromise recruitment of neutrophils and also innate immune surveillance (a phenomenon known as localized chemokine paralysis). In contrast, *A. actinomycetemcomitans* is more visible to the innate immune system and induces expression of IL-8, IL-6 and IL-1β from epithelial cells. Such differences in host epithelial cell responses may contribute to the different clinical outcomes associated with these organisms.

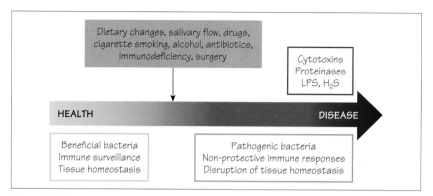

Figure 25.1 The status of periodontal tissues is a balance between factors contributing to health (left side) and factors contributing to disease (right side). External influences influence the flow from health towards disease.

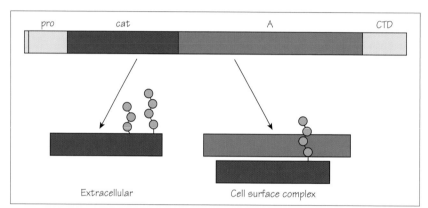

Figure 25.2 The major arginine (R) specific gingipain (RgpA proteinase) of *P. gingivalis* is expressed as a polyprotein comprised of the preprofragment (pro), the catalytic domain (cat), the adhesin/hemagglutinin domain (A) and the C-terminal domain (CTD) responsible for outer membrane translocation. The enzyme can be proteolytically processed into these domains and also processed within the A domain. Enzyme fragments can associate noncovalently in a variety of configurations and can be cell bound or extracellular. The protein is post translationally modified with glycan chains (green circles).

Table 25.1 Major virulence factors of common periodontal pathogens.

Virulence factor	Organism(s)	Action(s)
Leukotoxin Cytolethal distending toxin (CDT)	A. actinomycetemcomitans	Kills monocytes, neutrophils, and lymphocytes G2 arrest and apoptosis of lymphocytes
Proteases	P. gingivalis, P. intermedia, T. denticola, T. forsythia	Degrade matrix components, host cell receptors and immune effector molecules; alter vascular permeability; process bacteria surface adhesins; activate host MMPs, provide substrates for bacterial growth
LPS	Gram-negatives	Induction of inflammatory responses; osteoclast stimulation and bone resorption
Butyric acid and other short chain volatile fatty acids	P. gingivalis and other anaerobes	Host cell toxicity
Volatile sulfur compounds, ammonia and indole	P. gingivalis and other anaerobes	Host cell toxicity

Periodontal pathogens produce virulence factors that impact host immune responses, impinge upon tissue integrity and disrupt bone homeostasis (see Table 25.1). However, the onset of disease is determined by host factors and external influences, in addition to the periodontal microbiota (Figure 25.1).

Toxins

Periodontal pathogens generally do not produce potent exotoxins, although *Aggregatibacter actinomycetemcomitans* provides an exception. *A. actinomycetemcomitans* produces two major extracellular toxins, leukotoxin (LT) and cytolethal distending toxin (CDT). LT is a member of the RTX (repeats in toxin) family of pore forming hemolysins/leukotoxins expressed by a variety of pathogens. The leukotoxin operon consists of four genes involved in activation and transport of LT. LT targets only monocytes, neutrophils and a subset of lymphocytes from humans and some non-human primates that express the β2-integrin LFA-1. Cell death results from pore formation (high LT doses) or by apoptosis through mitochondrial perturbation (low LT doses). Strains of *A. actinomycetemcomitans* that are isolated from LAP lesions often have a re-arrangement in the promoter region of the LT gene that causes increased LT expression.

CDT is a heat labile cytotoxin homologous to toxins in *Escherichia coli* and some other Gram-negative pathogens. CDT induces G2 arrest of proliferating lymphocytes, as well as eukaryotic cell distension, actin rearrangements and apoptosis. CDT is a heterotrimer and the active sub-unit, CdtB, enters the cell while CdtA and CdtC remain associated with the cell surface.

Proteolytic enzymes

P. gingivalis produces a number of proteases with different specificities, although the best characterized are RgpA (Figure 25.2) and RgpB (arginine specific), and Kgp (lysine specific), collectively known as the gingipains and key virulence determinants. The primary function of *P. gingivalis* proteases is to provide peptides and heme (from host heme sequestering proteins) for the nutrition of this asaccharolytic, largely heme-dependent, organism. However, the broad specificity of these enzymes allows targeting of host structural proteins (e.g. collagens, fibronectin and laminin) and immune effector proteins (e.g. cytokines, antibodies, complement components, antimicrobial peptides and leukocyte surface receptors). Gingipains can activate the kallikrein cascade and cause the release of kinins with subsequent induction of vascular permeability which may allow systemic dissemination of *P. gingivalis*.

Gingipains also activate host matrix metalloproteinases (MMPs), particularly MMP-2 (gelatinase A-type IV collagenase), MMP-8 (neutrophil collagenase-2) and MMP-9 (gelatinase B-type IV collagenase). MMPs are a family of zinc-dependent proteinases secreted by many cell types that are activated by proteolysis and can degrade and modify matrix and basement membrane proteins in the periodontium. MMPs thus contribute to periodontal tissue destruction and failure of the periodontal lesion to heal. Gingipains can also degrade tissue inhibitors of MMPs (TIMPs).

RgpA and Kgp possess hemagglutinin (HagA) domains that mediate attachment to host cells. In addition, some *P. gingivalis* surface molecules such as FimA require protease activity for post-translational processing. Moreover, gingipain activity can expose previously hidden adhesin binding domains (cryptitopes) on host and bacterial proteins. *P. gingivalis* releases large numbers of membrane vesicles by evagination of the outer membrane. These vesicles possess adhesins and LPS present on the bacterial outer membrane, as well as entrapped periplasmic components. As vesicles contain proteases, one function may be to deliver proteolytic enzymes to the gingival tissues, which can also be penetrated by vesicles due to their small size.

Other proteinases produced by *P. gingivalis* include another group of cysteine proteases, aminopeptidases, prolyl dipeptidyl peptidase IV, and an endopeptidase with homology to endothelin-converting enzyme-like endopeptidase (PepO), important for epithelial cell invasion.

Prevotella intermedia produces several proteinases including a cysteine protease designated interpain A, trypsin-like serine proteases, and a dipeptidyl peptidase IV.

Treponema denticola produces a chymotrypsin-like protease CTLP, and a prolylalanine-specific protease PrtP. These proteases can form a complex along with Msp, a major OM protein with adhesive, porin and cytotoxic functions.

Tannerella forsythia produces an arginine specific cysteine protease (PrtH).

Bacterial components that impact alveolar bone

Loss of the alveolar bone that supports the tooth occurs in advanced periodontitis. Bacterial surface components can interfere with the balance between bone deposition by osteoblasts and resorption by osteoclasts. *P. gingivalis* LPS and fimbriae can stimulate osteoclasts and also induce the release from other cells of Interleukin (IL)-1β, PGE2 and TNFα, all of which are mediators of bone resorption. *A. actinomycetemcomitans* can activate osteoclasts through LPS and the molecular chaperone GroEL. Bone loss is discussed further in Chapter 26.

Other toxic products

P. gingivalis and other anaerobes produce butyric acid and other volatile fatty acids as metabolic end products. These short chain fatty acids are cytotoxic and can induce DNA fragmentation and apoptosis. Volatile sulfur compounds (hydrogen sulfide, methyl mercaptan and dimethyl sulfide), ammonia and indole produced by *P. gingivalis* and other anaerobes are also cytotoxic.

The immune response and periodontal bacteria

Table 26.1 Characteristics of major cytokines with relevance to periodontal disease

Cytokine	Cell source	Major biological activities
IL-1 α and β	Many cell types	Multiple pro-inflammatory functions, including stimulation of bone resorption, and MMP synthesis and release
IL-1ra	Macrophages, endothelial cells, keratinocytes	Receptor antagonist that inhibits action of IL-1
IL-4	Th2 lymphocytes	B cell proliferation, macrophage inhibition
IL-6	Many cell types	Multiple pro-inflammatory functions, similar to IL-1
IL-8	Macrophages, fibroblasts, PMNs, keratinocytes	Chemotactic for PMNs, T-cells and monocytes
IL-10	CD4/CD8 T cells, monocytes	Anti-inflammatory, inhibits macrophages and T-cells
IL-12	Macrophages, T and B cells	Stimulates Th1 lymphocytes
IL-13	T cells	B cell proliferation, macrophage inhibition
IL-17	T cells	Pro-inflammatory, stimulates bone resorption
TNF α and β	Macrophages, monocytes	Pro-inflammatory and can cause cell death
IFN-γ	NK cell and cytotoxic T-cells	Macrophage activation
MCP-1	Macrophages, monocytes, fibroblasts	Chemotactic for monocytes, T-cells and dendritic cells
MIP-1 α and β	Monocytes, fibroblasts, lymphocytes	Chemotactic for monocytes, T-cells and PMNs

Table 26.2 Genetic polymorphisms associated with periodontitis or periodontal health. Reproduced with permission from Lamont, Burne, Lantz, LeBlanc (eds) *Oral Microbiology and Immunology* (2006) ASM Press.

Polymorphism	Gene	Disease association
IL-1A (+4845) and IL-1B (+3954)	Interleukin-1 gene	Chronic periodontitis
TNF-alpha-308 allele 1	TNF-α gene	Chronic periodontitis
TNF-beta NcoI, ET-1 gene, and ACE gene insertion/deletion polymorphism	Lymphotoxin alpha (TNF-β), endothelin-1 (ET-1) and angiotensin-converting enzyme (ACE) genes	Chronic periodontitis
Fc gammaRIIIb-NA2 allotype	Fc receptor polymorphism	Chronic periodontitis
NAT2	N-acetyltransferase polymorphism	Chronic periodontitis
MMP-1 promoter polymorphism	Matrix metalloproteinase-1 gene	Chronic periodontitis
IL-1A (+4845) and IL-1B (+3954)	Interleukin-1 gene	Aggressive periodontitis
IL-1RN	Interleukin-1 receptor antagonist gene	Aggressive periodontitis (localized)
IL-4 promoter and intron polymorphisms	Interleukin-4 gene	Aggressive periodontitis
FcgammaRIIIb-NA2 allele (and possibly FcgammaRIIIa-158F)	Fc receptor gene polymorphisms	Aggressive periodontitis (generalized)
Gc locus chrom 4q	Unknown	Aggressive periodontitis (localized)
fMLP receptor	N-formyl peptide receptor polymorphisms	Aggressive periodontitis (localized)
VDR ApaI polymorphism	Vitamin D receptor polymorphism	Chronic and aggressive periodontitis (localized)
VDR gene Taq 1 polymorphism	Vitamin D receptor polymorphism	Aggressive periodontitis
HLA-A28 and HLA-B5	HLA haplotype	Periodontal health
FcgammaRIIIb-NA1	Fc receptor polymorphisms	Periodontal health

The initial periodontal lesion is characterized by an acute inflammatory response with vascular changes, collagen degradation and neutrophil infiltration. The host immune response is a double-edged sword that can be protective or destructive depending on context. A T-helper (Th)1 response develops in the early lesion with an increase in T lymphocyte infiltration, elevated loss of collagen and migration of epithelium down the root surface. However, interleukin (IL)-12 (Table 26.1) is produced which induces IFN-γ, which in turn activates macrophages and contributes to control of bacterial overgrowth. As the lesion becomes established, the levels of B lymphocytes, along with neutrophils, plasma cells and monocytes, begin to increase. Established and advanced lesions are consistent with Th2 responses, with production of IL-4, IL-10 and IL-13 and consequent antibody production. If the Th2 responses are insufficient to resolve or control the lesion there is subsequent additional connective tissue loss and osteoclastic alveolar bone loss. Recently, a novel subset of T-helper (Th) cells was identified that secretes several proinflammatory cytokines, including IL-17. IL-17 can support Th1 responses and promote neutrophil recruitment (protective responses) but may also stimulate osteoclastic bone resorption in combination with RANK-L (see below).

Importance of neutrophils

Neutrophils recruited through the gingival tissues create a barrier between the junctional epithelium and bacteria in the gingival crevice, and are thus the first line of innate defense against periodontal pathogens. Severe periodontitis, especially in young children, is frequently associated with congenital diseases that involve defects in neutrophil function such as leukocyte adhesion deficiency, Chediak–Higashi syndrome, Papillon–Lefèvre syndrome and chronic/cyclic neutropenia.

Not surprisingly, successful periodontal pathogens have evolved strategies to avoid neutrophil killing. *P. gingivalis* produces capsular polysaccharide that confers resistance to phagocytosis. Proteolytic degradation of opsonins (antibody and complement components) and neutrophil receptors by *P. gingivalis* also impedes phagocytosis. *P. gingivalis* can antagonize IL-8 secretion by epithelial cells following stimulation by commensal organisms, thus decreasing recruitment of neutrophils into the gingival crevice. In addition, neutrophils that remain in the gingival tissues and encounter bacteria can disgorge their lytic enzymes and contribute to tissue damage. *A. actinomycetemcomitans* produces Fc-binding proteins that inhibit phagocytosis by competing with neutrophils for binding to antibody opsonins. Once ingested, periodontal pathogens also show resistance to intracellular killing.

Innate immune sensing of periodontal bacteria

Cells of the innate host defense recognize periodontal bacteria, but there are mechanistic differences compared to commensal recognition, and a gradation of responses that may impact pathogenic potential.

Conserved bacterial structures (microbe associated molecular patterns, MAMPs), such as LPS are recognized by host cell pattern recognition receptors (PRRs), such as the toll-like receptors (TLRs), that initiate signaling events which control production of immune effector molecules such as cytokines (Chapter 8). The LPS from *P. gingivalis* is unusual in that it does not elicit potent inflammatory reactions in mice and can signal through both TLR2 and TLR4. *P. gingivalis* LPS displays lipid A structural heterogeneity, containing both penta and tetra-acylated lipid A structures, the ratios of which vary according to the concentration of hemin in the growth medium. The penta-acylated lipid A structures are TLR4 agonists, whereas tetra-acylated structures are TLR4 antagonists. The FimA fimbriae of *P. gingivalis* signal through TLR2 and TLR4, although other PRRs, such as CD14 and CD11b/CD18, are involved in recognition. Gingival epithelial cells respond poorly to the FimA fimbriae, as they do not express CD14, a co-receptor for TLR2. This may limit the inflammatory responses to fimbriated, invasive *P. gingivalis*. Recognition of *P. gingivalis* proteases by protease activated receptors (PARs) can also lead to the production of cytokines and antimicrobial β-defensins.

Tissue destruction and bone loss

Bone remodeling is controlled to a large extent by the balance and relative activities of RANK (receptor activator of NF-κB ligand), RANK-L (RANK ligand) and osteoprotegerin (OPG). RANK-L is expressed by osteoblasts and T-cells, and can be up-regulated by IL-1, TNF-α and PGE2, whereupon it induces osteoclast production and activation. In periodontal pockets the presence of inflammatory cytokines such as IL-1 and activated T-cells can lead to bone resorption through the RANK/RANK-L system. The effects of RANK-L are antagonized by the decoy receptor OPG which acts as a soluble neutralizing receptor. IL-1 and IL-6 can also act on osteoclasts directly to stimulate bone resorption.

The formation of immune complexes in tissue may also contribute to tissue destruction. It is important to remember that a periodontal lesion is in essence a wound that fails to heal. Organisms such as *P. gingivalis* can degrade fibrinogen/fibrin and dysregulate tissue repair by cleavage and activation of matrix metalloproteinases.

Genetic factors associated with periodontal disease

As periodontal diseases are multifactorial, a large number of host genetic factors may be associated with susceptibility to the disease (see Table 26.2). Genetic defects leading to neutrophil dysfunction are strongly associated with disease as discussed above. In aggressive periodontitis there are often high levels of IgG2 antibodies to bacterial carbohydrates. IgG2 is unique in that production is dependent on Th1 cytokines. While Th1 responses are known to be under genetic control, the genes involved in this condition have yet to be fully characterized.

Relationship between periodontal diseases and systemic health

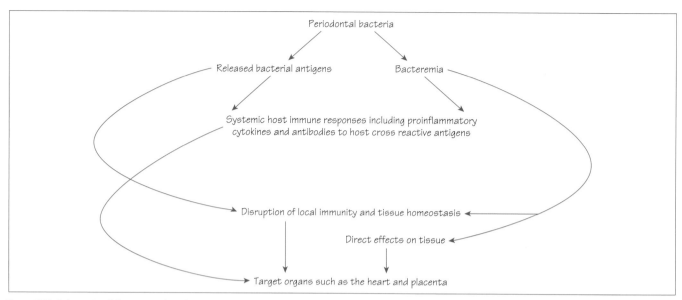

Figure 27.1 Schematic of the potential mechanisms linking periodontal status with systemic disease.

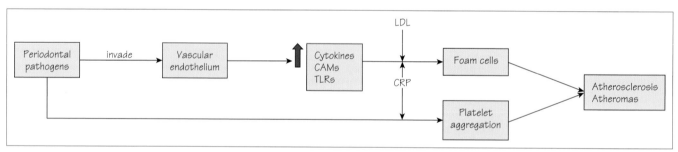

Figure 27.2 Possible connection between periodontal pathogens and cardiovascular disease.

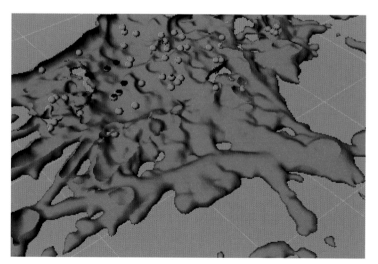

Figure 27.3 Cut away confocal microscopy image of a placental trophoblast cell (red) infected with P. gingivalis (green) and showing P. gingivalis is capable of internalizing within placental cells under experimental conditions.

While periodontal diseases are localized to the tissues supporting the teeth, evidence is emerging that periodontal infections and periodontal organisms are associated with serious systemic diseases such as cardiovascular disease, preterm delivery of low birth weight infants, pulmonary diseases, diabetes, osteoporosis and even Alzheimer's disease. Much of the evidence supporting these associations comes from epidemiological studies in which it is difficult to distinguish a causal relationship from an association resulting from a common predisposing factor. However, mechanistic bases for a direct causal link between periodontal diseases/organisms and systemic diseases is beginning to be established experimentally.

Pathogenic mechanisms – general principles

There are several broadly defined, and potentially interactive, mechanisms by which infections in the periodontal tissue could contribute to disease at remote sites (Figure 27.1). Periodontal bacteria and their antigens could initiate an inflammatory response in the periodontal tissues with systemic consequences. Moreover, bacteria and their products can gain access to the circulation during dental procedures such as scaling and root planing, or even after vigorous home care, especially in patients experiencing inflammation and tissue destruction such as occurs in periodontal disease. Once in the bloodstream, bacterial antigens could induce a systemic immune response. Periodontal bacteria in the blood could be carried to remote sites such as the placenta or heart tissues, either free in the circulation or within circulating cells such as monocytes or neutrophils, and initiate pathogenic processes at the remote sites. The ability of some periodontal bacteria, such as *P. gingivalis*, to resist both serum killing and oxygen-dependent killing within professional phagocytic cells would contribute to successful systemic dissemination. Finally, periodontal bacteria could initiate an autoimmune reaction, whereby bacterial antigens, such as heat shock proteins (HSPs) elicit a specific antibody that is cross-reactive with host molecules.

Cardiovascular disease (CVD)

Periodontal bacteria such as *P. gingivalis*, *T. forsythia*, *F. nucleatum*, *P. intermedia* and *A. actinomycetemcomitans* have been detected in carotid, coronary and aortic atheromatous plaques. It is important to note here, however, that detection was based on the presence of DNA, there has yet to be convincing evidence of live bacteria in atheromatous plaques. Nevertheless, *P. gingivalis* is capable of accelerating inflammatory plaque accumulation in the apolipoprotein E-knockout mouse model.

In vitro, *P. gingivalis* can invade and survive in endothelial cells, where it induces the secretion of proinflammatory cytokines and up-regulates expression of cell adhesion molecules (CAMs) and TLRs. Invasion of the vascular endothelium *in vivo* would thus be predicted to result in a pro-inflammatory, pro-thrombotic environment that is characteristic of atherosclerosis. In the presence of low-density lipoprotein (LDL), *P. gingivalis* can also induce foam cell formation by macrophages, a hallmark of early atherogenesis. Platelet aggregation can be induced by *P. gingivalis*, which could precede thrombo-embolic events (Figure 27.2).

A characteristic of both periodontal disease and CVD is elevated serum C-reactive protein (CRP). CRP can interfere with endothelial nitric oxide (NO) availability and is associated with the formation of a platelet-rich thrombus following plaque rupture or erosion, and with foam cell formation. CRP could thus provide a link between periodontal disease and CVD without the requirement for bacterial damage to vascular endothelium.

Adverse pregnancy outcomes

Periodontal diseases and organisms have been associated with pre-eclampsia and with preterm delivery of low birth weight infants (PLBW). *P. gingivalis* DNA has been detected in the amniotic fluid of pregnant women with threatened preterm labor, and *F. nucleatum* has been cultured from the amniotic fluid of women in preterm labor. In animal models both *P. gingivalis* and *F. nucleatum* are capable of reaching the placental tissues and inducing fetal death and PLBW. *P. gingivalis* is also capable of invading placental trophoblast cells in culture (Figure 27.3).

Pregnancy is maintained through a balance of cytokines and chemokines, proteases and hormones. Microbial infection can disrupt this balance and lead to PLBW. In the mouse model, *F. nucleatum* induces fetal death through stimulation of TLR4-mediated placental inflammatory responses.

Pulmonary infections

Periodontal bacteria and biofilm-derived aggregates that are inherently resistant to phagocytosis can be shed into the saliva and then aspirated into the lower respiratory tract and the lungs. Periodontal organisms may cause infection directly or cause local tissue damage that would facilitate infection by more traditional respiratory tract pathogens. Cytokines produced in response to periodontal bacteria may also reach the lungs, where they can stimulate local inflammatory processes that facilitate subsequent bacterial colonization and tissue damage.

Diabetes

While diabetes is a risk factor for periodontitis, conversely periodontal infection can result in increased cytokine production along with activation of acute-phase protein synthesis, and consequent insulin resistance. For example, TNF-α negatively regulates insulin signaling and glucose uptake, and IL-6 impairs the glucose-stimulated release of insulin from isolated pancreatic beta cells. Both IL-1β and IL-6 are capable of antagonizing insulin action.

Osteoporosis

Bone loss is a feature shared between periodontal disease and osteoporosis. The mechanisms by which periodontal bacterial can cause alveolar bone loss (Chapter 26), for example by RANK-L activation, could contribute to skeletal loss of bone mass and bone density.

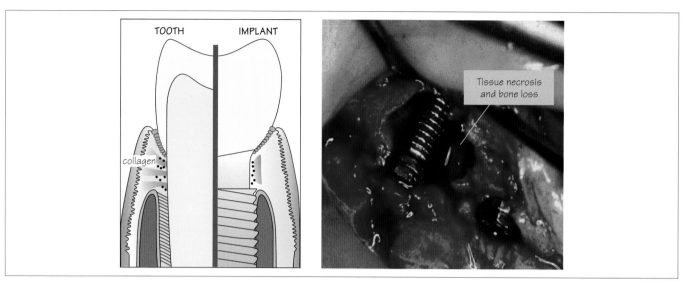

Figure 28.1 Diagrammatic vertical section comparison of tooth and implant showing collagen fiber distribution (left panel), and clinical photograph of a failed implant (right panel).

Table 28.1 Properties of titanium surfaces. Any titanium implant surface consists of an outer layer of titanium dioxide. The characteristics of this oxide layer may be divided into composition, topography and surface energy (wettability). All these affect biological reactions at the implant surface. Surface modifications may be used to improve bone bonding.

Surface topography	Implants come with roughened surfaces to improve bone bonding. Microsized topography can stimulate cell function and improve mechanical interlocking. Nanotopography is being developed to target specific cell functions for better control of cell behaviour
Composition	Calcium and phosphate (elements of hydroxyapatitie) may be incorporated into implant surfaces to match bone tissue (biomimetic). Crystallinity (the way Ti and O atoms are arranged) is also believed to affect implant performance
Wettabiliy	The wettability, or hydrophilicity, of an implant surface is very important for protein and cell adhesion. Some commercially available implants are kept in isotonic solution
Functionally loaded	Next generation implants may be more intelligent with biological molecules such as growth factors or specific proteins incorporated onto the surfaces (functionally loaded surface). The ability to slowly release such biological factors from an implant inserted into bone is also desirable

Table 28.2 Organisms most commonly isolated from peri-implantitis lesions

Microorganisms associated with peri-implantitis
Porphyromonas gingivalis
Prevotella intermedia
Fusobacterium species
Aggregatibacter actinomycetemcomitans
Staphylococcus aureus
Enterococcus faecalis
Candida albicans

Dental implants are becoming more common in the clinical setting. They are used in the repair of accidental damage to the jaw or dentition, or to replace teeth lost through decay or affected by trauma. In the most routine surgical procedure, a titanium (Ti) screw barrel is inserted into alveolar bone, usually into a vacant tooth socket. There is then a period of convalescence for the subject when the titanium implant is allowed to become stably incorporated into alveolar bone. This process is termed osseo-integration and is crucial to the success of the implant. A suitably shaped and colored artificial tooth is then screwed into the titanium barrel (see Figure 28.1). Because bone growth is stimulated by mechanical force or load, there has to be mechanical load applied to the implant over a period of time. Techniques being developed to speed up this process, by providing high loads at early stages, are risky. Implants should never be inserted into weakened alveolar bone or at inflamed sites. Teeth that have been lost as a result of periodontitis are not substitutable by implants because the implant will generally fail to osseo-integrate.

Osseo-integration

There are two important classes of cells involved in bone production and turnover. Osteoblasts are fibroblast-like cells that produce collagen and are responsible for bone cell development and mineralization. Osteoclasts are derived from cells in the bone marrow. They regulate bone production by removing the mineralized matrix, termed resorption, and remodeling bone structure. Titanium surfaces that allow bone cells (osteoblasts) to attach to them would be better integrated into the bone (Table 28.1). Growth factors and other compounds can improve the attachment or differentiation of osteoblasts growing in association with titanium. Currently, it is thought that oxidized titanium surfaces are more effective for cell attachment. Regular patterned arrays of only micrometer dimensions may be machined across the surface of titanium to promote osteoblast attachment and spreading.

Implant structure

There are differences in tissue structure of the mucosa surrounding the implant, compared with that surrounding the tooth root. In the latter (Figure 28.1 left panel) bundles of collagen fibers radiate out into the cementum of the root. With implants, collagen fiber bundles run parallel to the surface of the implant (Figure 28.1). Also, there are differences in composition of the connective tissue. The connective tissue of the mucosa around the implant has high collagen content. It is more similar to scar tissue and contains a much reduced blood supply. This contributes to a general decrease in immune function and to an increase in susceptibility to peri-implant infections.

Peri-implantitis

This condition refers to microbial infections that occur following implant surgery. Infection may be early after surgery, shown by redness, inflammation, discharge and rapid loss of bone. However, disease may take much longer to develop, resulting in alveolar bone resorption and rejection of the implant (Figure 28.1 right panel). The inflammation and inflammatory process goes deeper and faster around an implant compared to an adjacent natural tooth. Once this happens it is unlikely that a subsequent implant will be successful. The disease is very much like periodontal disease, but is acute and more destructive.

Bacteria associated with peri-implantitis

In disease conditions, the bacteria associated with the natural tooth or implant are very similar. They include *P. gingivalis*, *Prevotella intermedia*, *Fusobacterium* and *A. actinomycetemcomitans*. However, there is often a much higher incidence of motile spirochetes at implant sites. Other microorganisms involved with infections at implant sites are varied. *Staphylococcus aureus*, enteric bacteria, such as *E. faecalis* and *Candida albicans* are commonly often found in peri-implant lesions (Table 28.2). By contrast, implants surrounded by healthy tissue demonstrate a microbiota associated with periodontal health. All peri-implant infections have a common feature: if they are not treated the infection leads to loss of the implant.

Asepsis and treatment

Dental implants are becoming increasingly important in prosthodontic rehabilitation. Bacterial infections, however, can induce bone loss and jeopardize clinical success. One area of concern is that the implants are properly sterile before insertion. Recently it has been demonstrated that infra-red CO_2 laser light is suitable for the decontamination of exposed implant surfaces. Another treatment regimen, photodynamic therapy (PDT), involves the use of a non-toxic dye (a photosensitizer) and low-intensity laser light. These combine to create singlet oxygen molecules that are lethal to certain bacteria. Laser treatment is best combined with surgical opening of the implant site for cleaning and disinfecting the local defect. In this way, photodynamic therapy can be used successfully to decontaminate the implant surface.

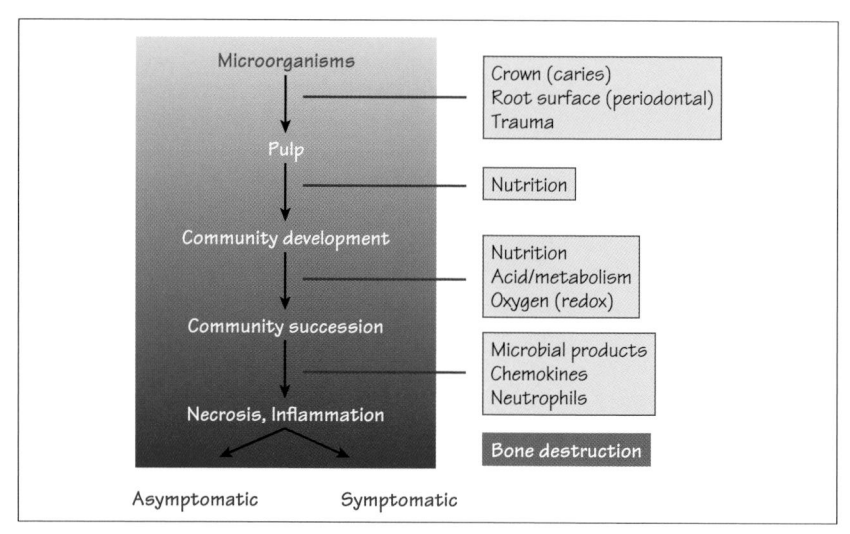

Figure 29.1 Course of endodontic infection following entry of microorganisms into the pulp.

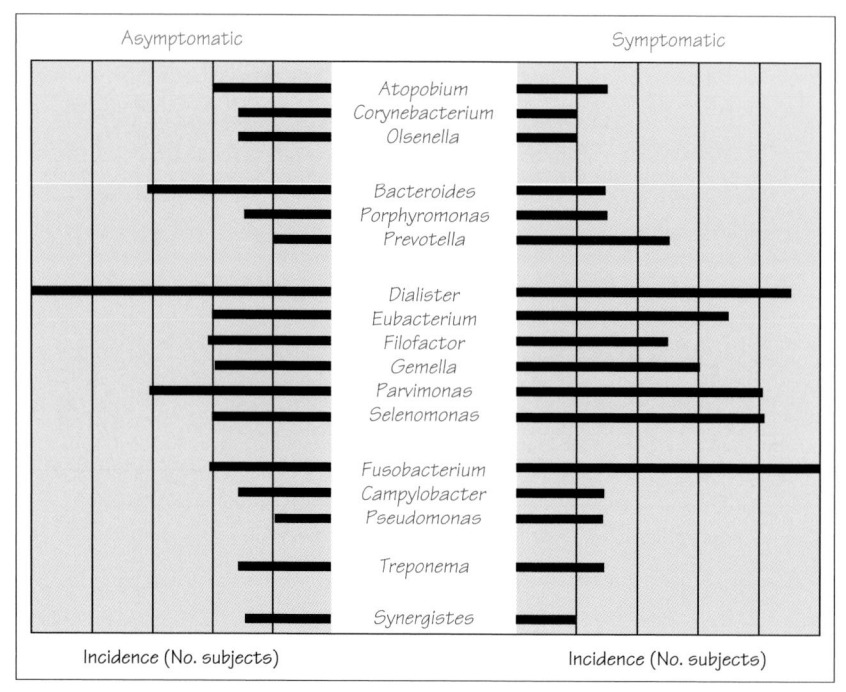

Figure 29.2 Microorganisms recovered from asymptomatic and symptomatic root canals.

Table 29.1 Cultivable microorganisms recovered from infected root canals.

Most prevalent cultivable taxa from infected root canals include:
- Fusobacterium nucleatum
- Porphyromonas gingivalis
- Pseudoramibacter alactolyticus
- Parvimonas micra (P. micros)
- Streptococcus mitis
- Streptococcus oralis/sanguinis/intermedius

Dominated by anaerobic bacteria
Most prevalent genus is Streptococcus

Table 29.2 Species diversity in infected root canals.

Phylotypes common to asymptomatic and symptomatic endodontic infections:
- Dialister, Fusobacterium, Prevotella, Veillonella

Most common organisms detected by molecular studies independently of symptoms:
- Porphyromonas endodontalis, Filofactor alocis, Porphyromonas gingivalis, Tannerella forsythia, Pseudoramibacter alactolyticus

Archaea (Methanobrevibacter) convert H_2 to methane
Root canal samples from asymptomatic infections show higher diversity of species

Endodontic infections refer to those that occur within the tooth pulp, root canal system or at the root apex (Figure 29.1). Normally the pulp and root canal system are sterile. However, bacteria may enter through cracks around restorations, areas of exposed dentin and possibly microfracture, or through trauma to the tooth. There is also a theory that microbes present transiently in the circulatory system could become lodged within the apical region of the root and cause abscess formation. One of the major areas of debate is how exactly complex populations of bacteria form inside the root canal system. However, there is good evidence that oral bacteria may penetrate the dentinal tubules.

Dentinal tubules

Dentinal tubules are present within and across dentin. They are produced during dentin formation by odontoblast migration. The tubules are wider at the pulpal side (approx. 2.5 μm) and contain more collagen fibers. The tubules are narrower at the dentino-enamel junction side (approx. 0.9 μm) and more calcified. Dentinal fluid (containing albumin, transferrin, tenascin and protoglycans) is present within the tubules, giving dentin a permeability which increases the sensation of pain. Bacteria may penetrate these tubules if dentin is exposed, or invade the tubules from the pulpal side. Bacteria present within tubules are hard to eliminate. They are well protected from defense molecules and from antiseptics used in endodontic surgery. Bacterial infection affects the hydrostatic pressure within tubules, increasing the sensitivity to hot or cold liquids or food.

Bacterial invasion of dentin

The populations of bacteria present in long-term root canal and pulpal infections (pulpitis) are complex. In laboratory experiments, dentin is most quickly infected by bacteria that are not necessarily main components of the root canal microbiota. For example, *S. mutans* and *S. gordonii* readily infect dentinal tubules, and can penetrate to depths of 0.2 mm or more over several days. *P. gingivalis* cannot penetrate dentinal tubules in pure culture, but can invade in combination with streptococci to which it attaches. Thus, direct microbial interactions may be important in generating root canal microbiota.

Microbiota of endodontic infections

Studies of the endodontic bacteria have relied heavily on anaerobic cultivation techniques to identify the components. However, molecular approaches have considerably improved the analyses, showing that some initial interpretations were incorrect. For example, in many cases *Entercococcus faecalis* was isolated as a component of early root canal infections. It is clear now that this organism, whilst found in some cases, is not the major pathogen that it was believed to be. Somewhere between 50 and 60 taxa are found associated with endodontic infections. The most prevalent cultivable taxa from root canals are *F. nucleatum*, *P. gingivalis*, *Pseudoramibacter alactolyticus*, *Parvimonas micra (Peptostreptococcus micros)*, *S. mitis*, *S. intermedius*, other streptococci and *Candida*. The microbiota is dominated by anaerobic bacteria, but the most prevalent genus is *Streptococcus* (Table 29.1). Molecular methods reveal that there are many bacteria present that are uncultivable, including *Treponema*, *Filofactor alocis*, *Dialister pneumosintes*, *Dialister invisus*, *Olsenella uli* and *Olsenella profusa*. The most common organisms detected by molecular studies, independently of symptoms, are *Porphyromonas endodontalis*, *Filofactor alocis*, *P. gingivalis*, *T. forsythia*, and *P. alactolyticus*. Archaea are also present, e.g. *Methanobrevibacter* that converts H_2 to methane (Table 29.2). About 50% of the bacteria will not grow on artificial media. This may be due to lack of essential nutrients, medium toxicity, or dependence upon another species. Primary infections have been found to contain 10–30 species of bacteria. However, persistent infections contain fewer species. No single species of bacterium is recognized as a pathogen.

Symptomatic versus asymptomatic

There has been considerable debate about whether or not different species of bacteria are associated with symptomatic (pain) or asymptomatic conditions. Phylotypes common to both asymptomatic and symptomatic endodontic infections are *Dialister*, *Fusobacterium*, *Prevotella* and *Veillonella*. There is, however, some tentative data suggesting that the incidence of *Fusobacterium* and *Eubacterium* is higher in symptomatic conditions (Figure 29.2).

Treatment

Patients with acute pain are often given antibiotics, such as amoxicillin and metronidazole. However, the bacteria are so protected within the pulpal region that antibiotics are often of no benefit. Root canals are cleared of pulp and debris by the clinician, and characteristically irrigated with sodium hypochlorite, and a calcium hydroxide paste applied. Both these regimens are anti-bacterial, although some organisms, e.g. *E. faecalis* are more resistant. Because sodium hypochlorite also damages host tissues, other irrigants or sterilants have been promoted. One of these is ozone, which is bactericidal, but it is rapidly inactivated by organic matter.

Host factors in endodontic infections

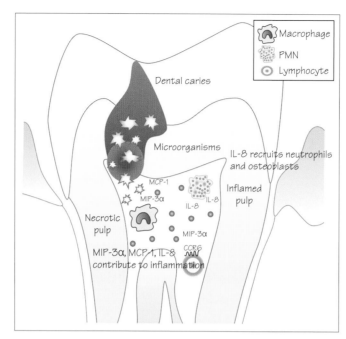

Figure 30.1 *Generation of host immune responses to microorganisms within the pulp. Reproduced with permission from Silva TA et al. Chemokines in oral inflammatory diseases: apical periodontitis and periodontal disease. Journal of Dental Research (2007); 86: 306–319.*

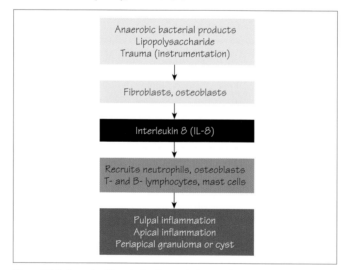

Figure 30.2 Key role of Interleukin 8 in endodontic infections.

Table 30.1 Cytokines in apical periodontitis.

Roles of individual cytokines not known

Elevated IL-8/CXCL8, MIP-3a/CCL20, MCP-1/CCL-2 characteristic of inflamed pulp

MIP-3a/CCL20 produced by macrophages

IL-8 activity in cyst epithelial lining

Balance of cytokines, chemokines regulate migration, proliferation and matrix synthesis

Evaluation of lesion progression, e.g. active or healing

Clinical symptoms of endodontic infections result from inflammation of the pulp in response to microbial challenge. In these respects, endodontic infections are very much like periodontal infections. Pulpal infection can progress to the periapical region and generate alveolar bone destruction and chronic apical periodontitis. The immunology and host innate responses to microbial challenge are just beginning to be understood. Essentially, chemokines are generated in response to bacterial infection of pulp. These contribute to inflammation and recruit ostoeblasts and neutrophils. The pulpal inflammation may then progress to the apical region (Figure 30.1).

Pulpal infections

The inflammatory and immune responses that are initiated by bacteria are generated in order to protect the host against infection. The persistence of a local chronic response alters the protective role of inflammatory cells and produces deleterious effects. Development of periodontal disease is associated with progression of inflammatory cell infiltrate into the deeper periodontal tissues. Dental pulp is normally protected from the bacteria of the oral cavity by the presence of enamel and dentin. Exposure of dental pulp to bacteria as a result of dental caries, fractures, or operative procedures triggers a pulpal inflammatory response. Severe pulpitis, which occurs often as a result of dental caries, is characterized by the presence of a major inflammatory infiltrate. However, little is understood about how these cells are recruited into dental pulp lesions. Pulp cells are able to respond to bacteria and toxins through chemokine production. A high concentration of interleukin 8 (IL-8), a major chemo-attractant of PMNs, has been detected in pulps that have been diagnosed with irreversible pulpitis. Normal pulps show only weak, or no, IL-8.

Periapical abscesses

In inflamed pulp the chemokines MIP-3a, IL-8 and MCP-1 contribute to inflammatory cell infiltration (Table 30.1). Progression of pulpal inflammation to the periapical region leads to adaptive and innate immune responses. The outcome is periapical alveolar bone destruction and lesion formation. Combinations of bacteria appear to be more effective inducers of bone resorption than single species. Chronic apical periodontitis is referred to as periapical granuloma and can evolve to produce a periapical cyst. The main components of these lesions are PMNs, macrophages, T and B lymphocytes, mast cells, osteoclasts and osteoblasts. Chemokines are key elements in the formation of granulomas, and their production is elicited by bacteria. The predominantly anaero-bic microbiota of the root canals (*P. gingivalis*, *P. endodontalis*, *Prevotella intermedia*, etc.) are all able to induce the production of IL-8 by pulp fibroblasts, and MIP-1α and MIP-1β by neutrophils. A positive association between IL-8 levels and painful symptoms has been reported. Chemokine production in periapical lesions may also be stimulated by trauma, injury from instrumentation or irritation from chemicals used in endodontics (Figure 30.2). Often, chemical and mechanical preparation of the root canal, in conjunction with filling of the root canal system, leads to elimination of an infection and healing of the periapical tissues. In some instances, however, apical periodontitis does not respond to treatment. It is thought that this is due to the anatomical complexity of root canals, which makes the elimination of microorganisms difficult. Host factors must also function suitably to effect repair. Thus, migration of lymphocytes, neutrophils and mononuclear cells is essential for the periapical tissue response.

Repair and angiogenesis

Chemokines are considered to be important for the recruitment of sub-populations of leukocytes. Cytokines can also help repair tissue and promote angiogenesis. Expression of MIP-1α has been linked to enhanced macrophage influx, angiogenic activity and collagen production. The higher expression of chemokines, e.g. MCP-1, CCR3, CCR5 and CXCR1 in cysts compared with granulomas may be significant in the development of granulomas to cysts. Chemokines might be useful for evaluating the progression of periapical lesions. It could be determined whether the lesions are active or healing by sampling through the root canal before obturation. This knowledge may provide new means for controlling apical periodontitis.

Resistant bacteria

Survival of bacteria within periapical tissues is probably the reason for endodontic treatment failures. The periapical microbiota in these instances is usually dominated by Gram-positive organisms and is different from the microbiota that appears to respond to treatment. Resistant organisms include *Streptococcus*, *Staphylococcus*, *Bacillus*, *Pseudomonas*, *Enterococcus* and *Candida*. The organisms become adapted to live in the environment and may be surrounded by matrix as in a biofilm. The microorgansims responsible for long-term infections may not necessarily be conventional oral bacteria. For example, *Psuedomonas aeruginosa* has been found frequently to be an associated agent. Often, antibiotics such as metronidazole and carbenicillin, which may be effective in periodontal control, are ineffective in eliminating periapical infections.

31 Infective endocarditis

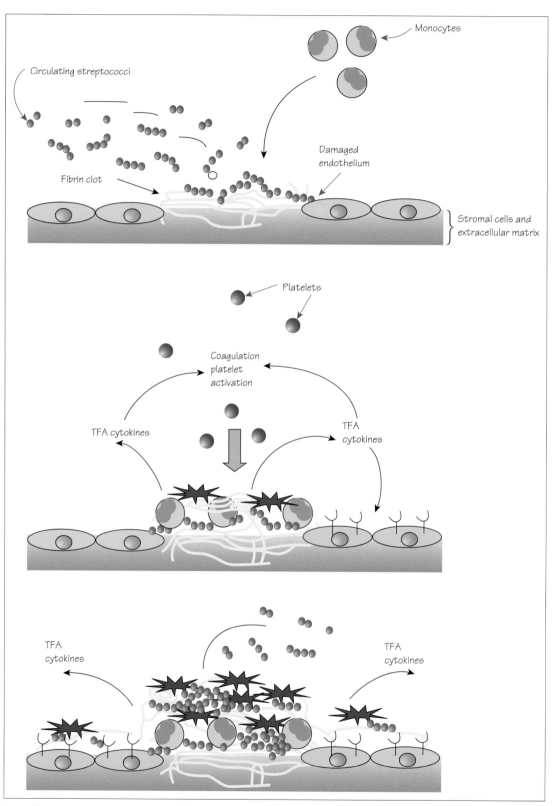

Figure 31.1 *Growth of a thrombotic vegetation following bacterial attachment to damaged endothelial sites. Reproduced with permission from Moreillon P, Que Y-A Infective endocarditis. Lancet (2004), 363: 139–149.*

Endocarditis is an inflammation of the inner layer of the heart, characterized by formation of a vegetation. This is a mass of platelets, fibrin, some inflammatory cells and microorganisms. Infective endocarditis (IE) has a low incidence rate (1 in 10–100,000, depending upon population) but high mortality. In the past, IE was divided into sub-acute (low virulence proceeding over weeks or months) or acute (a sudden illness over days or weeks). However, this terminology is no longer used. Altered blood flow around the heart valves is a risk factor for infective endocarditis. The valves may be damaged from surgery, autoimmune disease (e.g. rheumatic fever), or simply from old age. Vegetations result from bacteremia, the presence of bacteria in the blood. This occurs quite easily, for example by vigorous tooth brushing, also from urinary tract infections and in IV drug users. The latter tend to get their right side valves infected because the veins injected go into the right side of the heart. In rheumatic heart disease the aortic and mitral valves are affected in the left side of the heart. It is also important to distinguish between native valve and prosthetic valve disease. Early prosthetic valve endocarditis usually is due to operative or post-operative bacterial contamination.

Bacteria in IE

The viridans streptococci (most commonly *S. sanguinis*), and related but unidentified oral streptococci, account for about 50% of IE cases in the developing world. The streptococcal-like genera include *Gemella*, *Granulicatella* and *Abiotrophia*. Approximately another 30% of cases are due to *S. aureus*, and these develop more rapidly as *S. aureus* is more virulent than oral streptococci. *Enterococcus faecalis* and *Enterococcus faecium* (Lancefield group D organisms) are also frequent agents of IE, accounting for about 10% of cases. They are often derived from urinary tract infections and are hospital acquired. The most important diagnosis for IE is blood culture of the microorganisms combined with results of echocardiography. However, culture-negative endocarditis accounts for about 10% of cases, and some of the pathogens responsible are *Aspergillus*, *Brucella*, *Coxiella* and *Chlamydia*.

Mechanism of vegetation formation

Formation of a vegetation begins by bacteria becoming established at a site of injury on a heart valve, or on the wall of a blood vessel (endothelial site). Bacteria interact with the fibrin-platelet clot, and with fibronectin or collagen exposed as a result of damage. In experimental animals the fibronectin-binding proteins FnBPA and FnBPB are necessary for *S. aureus* to cause IE. Once attached to the host site (see Figure 31.1), bacteria interact with blood platelets by transiently trapping them and causing them to roll. This mimics the natural system for blood vessel repair whereby endothelial damage is recognized by von Willebrand factor, which is activated by collagen and traps circulating platelets. Tissue factor (TFA) is involved in the formation of thrombin. Once platelets are trapped by the bacteria, fibrinogen accumulates and is converted by thrombin protease to fibrin. The platelets become activated and aggregate in close association with the bacteria to form a thrombotic vegetation.

Bacterial virulence factors

Fibronectin binding proteins in *S. aureus*, and matrix-binding proteins in *E. faecalis* are involved in IE. However, platelet interactions are important in the generation of thrombi. *S. sanguinis* and *S. gordonii* produce cell-surface proteins GspB/Hsa (and homologs are present in other streptococci) that specifically recognize sialic acid residues on human platelet receptors. The sialic acid present on platelet glycoprotein Ib (GPIb) is bound by this streptococcal protein, effectively providing the means by which platelets are trapped in the circulation. GPIb is the platelet receptor recognized by von Willebrand factor, so the bacteria mimic the activity of a host protein. Subsequently, other proteins present on the bacterial cell surface may induce platelet aggregation and activation. This occurs in conjunction with binding of fibrinogen (*S. aureus* ClfA protein binds fibrinogen) and with antibody reacting with the platelet Fc receptor. Other specific virulence factors have been identified in streptococci and staphylococci. The metal ion binding proteins FimA, ScaA and SloA in viridans streptococci are virulence factors for IE, as is polysaccharide production by *S. mutans*. Animals vaccinated with SloA are partially protected against *S. mutans* induced IE, suggesting that vaccination of high risk groups could be beneficial.

Antibiotics in IE

In the past, bacteremia caused by certain dental procedures, e.g. tooth extraction was thought to be significant in IE. Consequently, patients with heart problems were given antibiotic prophylaxis in case of infection. This practice has now ceased in many countries as there is no firm evidence that dental treatment increases the risk for IE any more than simply brushing or flossing teeth. For subjects presenting with IE, high dose antibiotics are administered by the intravenous route, often for long periods (up to six weeks). This maximizes the diffusion of antibiotics into the vegetations. Viridans group streptococci are highly sensitive to pencillin, whereas treating for *S. aureus* might require oxacillin or vancomycin. Fungal endocarditis requires anti-fungal treatment such as with amphotericin B.

32 Oral mucosal, bone and systemic infections

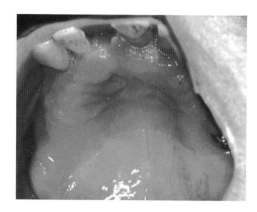

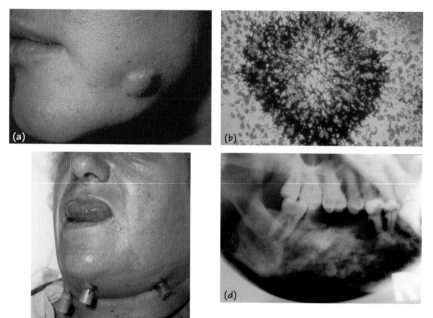

Figure 32.1 Denture stomatitis on upper palate. Inflammation has occurred underneath the denture and is delineated by the red line.

Figure 32.2 Examples of odontogenic infections associated with oral bacteria. (a) cyst typical of actinomycosis; (b) rosette of *Actinomyces israelii* within cyst; (c) Ludwig's angina, showing external drains for inflammatory exudate, and raised tongue due to swelling of sub-lingual space; (d) osteomyelitis of the jaw.

Table 32.1 Oral microbe-associated infections, the etiologic agents and their origins.

Disease	Agent(s)	Origin
Mucosal lesions	S. aureus, enterococci, Neisseria, enteric bacteria, Candida	Oral colonizers or transients
Halitosis	Fusobacterium, Porphyromonas, Prevotella, Treponema, Eubacterium	Oral colonizers of tongue
Angular cheilitis	S. aureus, C. albicans	Oral colonizers or transients
Osteomyelitis of lower jaw	S. aureus, Pseudomonas	Dentoalveolar
Actinomycosis	Actinomyces israelii	Oral colonizer
Osteonecrosis	Polymicrobial including A. israelii	Oral colonizers or transients
Submucosal abscess	Polymicrobial	Oral
Brain abscess	Polymicrobial (periodontal microflora)	Periodontitis, periapical abscess
Chronic sinusitis	Ill defined	Periodontitis
Ludwig's angina	Polymicrobial (periodontal microbiota and viridans streptococci)	Periapical abscess, periodontitis, dental caries
Lung abscess	Actinomyces, Aggregatibacter, Prevotella	Periodontitis
Chronic obstructive lung	Pseudomonas aeruginosa	Oral transient
Prosthetic joint infection	Peptostreptococcus, Streptococcus	Periodontitis, periapical abscess
Chronic meningitis	Streptococcus	Periapical abscess, dental caries
Acute meningitis	Neisseria meningitidis, S. sanguinis	Periodontitis, endodontic therapy

Most of oral microbiology is concerned with infections of the teeth and gums leading to dental caries and periodontal disease. There are, however, many disease conditions of the oral mucosa and submucosa and systemic conditions, in addition to infective endocarditis, that may result from mobilization of oral microbiota components. Infections of the mucosa are more usually associated with transient oral bacteria. For example, staphylococci are found in the saliva of approximately 30% individuals, but they are considered transients rather than components of the resident oral microbiota. Likewise Gram-positive enterococci, and Gram-negative facultatively anaerobic rods, e.g. *E. coli*, *Klebsiella*, *Pseudomonas*, are transient bacteria in saliva. However, all these microorganisms can play a significant role in oral and respiratory tract infections of a compromised host.

Mucosal infections

Epithelial cell desquamation prevents accumulation of microorganisms upon epithelial surfaces on the palate, on the floor of the mouth and on the inside buccae. By contrast, the dorsum of the tongue provides a surface of papillae and taste buds for rich microbial biofilms to develop. Halitosis can be caused by bacteria on the tongue processing proteins into: volatile sulfur compounds such as hydrogen sulfide, methyl mercaptan and dimethyl sulfide; phenyls, such as indole, skatole and pridine; diamines, such as putrescine and cadaverine; or short chain fatty acids such as butyric acid and propionic acid. Halitosis can also be caused by extra-oral and systemic conditions. The most common mucosal lesions are stomatitis (Figure 32.1) and angular cheilitis (see Chapter 33) which involve combinations of *Candida* fungi and bacteria. Microbes associated with lesions include *S. aureus*, enterococci, enterobacteriacae and *Candida* (see Table 31.1). Factors that pre-dispose to mucosal infections include mechanical injury, associated with impaired function of the tongue or impaired salivary flow, inadequate oral hygiene especially of dentures and faulty restorations, and systemic influences such as chemotherapeutics, impaired immune function and malnutrition.

Submucosal and bone infections

Submucosal infections, caused by bacteria penetrating the epithelial barrier and entering underlying tissues, usually form abscesses (Figure 32.2). Most of these infections are polymicrobial and anaerobic. In individuals with normal immune function, submucosal infections only occur as a result of local predisposing factors. These include necrotic pulp, dental calculus, deep periodontal pockets and soft tissue damage. A complication of subepithelial infections is spreads to the head and neck. Osteomyelitis may occur in the lower jaw and has similar microbiology to periodontal or endodontal conditions. Actinomycosis is a specific infection, developing in the head and neck and affecting the lower jaw. Infected root canals provide the point of entry for *Actinomyces* bacteria, which set up what is commonly a chronic infection. A hard swelling develops, often with formation of a granuloma in which aggregates of *Actinomyces* cells appear as grains (so called 'sulfur granules'). *Actinomyces israelii* is the most commonly isolated species from human actinomycosis. Osteonecrosis of the jaw is associated with bisphosphonates, a class of drugs that inhibit osteoclasts and bone resorption, and are used in the prevention and treatment of osteoporosis. Osteonecrosis of the jaw often follows high-dose intravenous administration as is used for some cancer patients. *A. israelii* is associated with this condition, most likely in a mixed biofilm with other oral organisms such as *Fuosbacterium*, *Treponema* and yeasts.

Oral manifestations of systemic infections

Many human infections at other body sites may manifest in changes within the oral cavity. These can be important in the diagnosis of non-oral conditions. For example, both gonorrhea and syphilis cause oral lesions, either as grayish areas on the tongue and soft palate (gonorrhea) or as hard chancres (primary syphilis) or small gray mucous syphilitic patches (secondary). Lepromas, containing *Mycobacterium leprae*, form on the tongue and palates in immunocompromised subjects with leprosy. Tularemia, caused by *Francisella tularensis*, is a febrile illness transmitted by insects into humans from rodents and birds. In humans, initial infections occur on the fingers, or as oral lesions, as a result of eating infected meat. These lesions can be mistaken for syphilitic lesions. Many forms of mucosal lesion indicate some degree of immune dysfunction that may be localized or systemic.

Systemic manifestations of oral infections

Brain infections and disorders may occur secondarily to bacteremias derived from the oral cavity. *Streptococcus*, *Peptostreptococcus*, *Prevotella* and *Fusobacterium* have all been isolated from brain abscesses. Periodontal and periapical infections can spread into tissues surrounding the oral cavity leading to maxillary sinusitis, Ludwig's angina and fascial plane infections. Lung abscesses may be caused by aspiration of salivary or dental plaque bacteria. Acute respiratory infections may follow aspiration during dental treatment. Chronic obstructive pulmonary infections in cystic fibrosis patients may be caused by mucoid variant strains of *Pseudomonas aeruginosa* colonizing the buccal mucosa and being aspirated into the lungs. Prosthetic joint infections involving *Peptostreptococcus* and viridans streptococci can occur following systemic spread. Chronic meningitis has been related to periapical abscesses and dental caries. A case of osteomyelitis of the ulna caused by *P. gingivalis* has been reported. For more on systemic conditions possibly associated with periodontal pathogens see Chapter 27.

33 Candida albicans and fungal infections

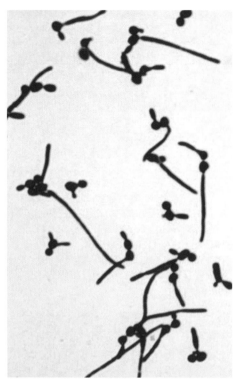

Figure 33.1 Image of *Candida albicans* showing yeast cells (blastospores), pseudohyphae (small projections) and true hyphal filaments.

Table 33.1 *Candida species infections in humans.*

Superficial candidiasis	Disseminated candidiasis
Cutaneous	Candidemia
Perianal	Chronic disseminated
Submammary	Urogenital
Granuloma	Endocarditis
Mucocutaneous	Meningitis
Glossitis	Encephalitis
Stomatitis	Phlebitis
Cheilitis	
Bronchitis	
Esophagitis	
Pneumonia	
Enteritis	

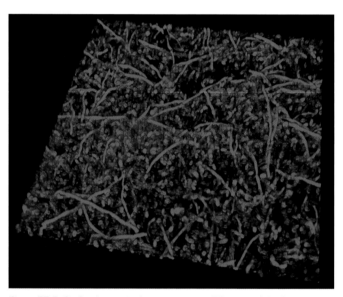

Figure 33.3 Confocal scanning laser microscope 3D image of *C. albicans* biofilm formed on salivary pellicle, showing hyphal filaments intertwined with yeast forms.

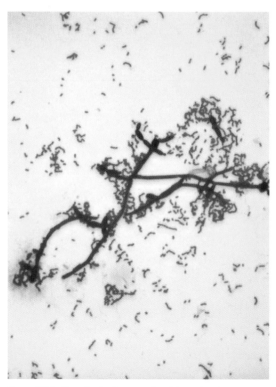

Figure 33.2 Co-adhesion between *Candida* and oral streptococci.

Candida albicans is found as part of the human microbiota of the digestive tract, which includes the mouth. There are approximately 200 different species of *Candida* yeasts. *C. albicans* accounts for 75% of all fungal infections of humans. Up to 40% of healthy adults carry *C. albicans* in their mouths. In general, *Candida* grows and survives as a commensal. However, a slight modification of the host defenses, or of the commensal microbiota, can provide an opportunity for *Candida* to breach the protective barriers and become pathogenic. *C. albicans* is a good example of an opportunistic pathogen. It is a pleiomorphic (many forms) fungus, growing as an oval shaped budding yeast, or as pseudohyphae or true hyphae (Figure 33.1). The transition from yeast form to hyphal form is one of the many characteristics associated with virulence. Other microbial components involved in pathogenesis include: adhesins, such as HWP1 (hyphal wall protein), which promote colonization; hydrolytic enzymes, e.g. proteases, phospholipases, that cause tissue destruction; and molecules like CR3-like receptor and HSP90 (heat shock protein) that modulate immune system functions. Pathogenesis is facilitated by breakdown of host immunity by immunodeficiency diseases or by iatrogenic factors. The latter include chemical or physical therapeutic interventions that weaken the defenses at various levels.

C. albicans infections (Table 33.1)

Infections caused by *Candida* may be superficial or systemic. The superficial infections include those of the cutaneous or mucocutaneous tissues (Table 33.1). Systemic infections, which have high mortality rates, may involve multiple organs. Mucocutaneous candidiasis occurs in subjects who have cellular immune deficiency, are immunosuppressed, or have their protective commensal microbiota disturbed. The incidence of systemic candidiasis has increased over the past two decades, and *Candida* species such as *albicans*, *dubliniensis*, *tropicalis*, *parapsilosis* and *glabrata* are significant nosocomial (hospital-acquired) pathogens. The increase is due mainly to more invasive surgical techniques, the growing use of prosthetic devices such as intravascular catheters, and new drug therapies. Prosthetic devices provide new surfaces for microbial colonization, and *C. albicans* is efficient at forming robust biofilms.

Denture stomatitis

This is a *Candida* infection of the oral mucosa caused by a close-fitting upper denture. This cuts off the mucosa from the normal protective and lubricatory properties of saliva. It is rarely seen under a lower denture because this is more mobile and salivary flow is usually unrestricted. *Candida* hyphal forms may be seen microscopically as having grown between the denture and mucosa. Bacteria are also present in this condition, such as *Streptococcus*, but also *S. aureus* and *E. coli*, and may enhance inflammation in the palatal mucosa.

Angular cheilitis

This is frequently associated with denture stomatitis and involves leakage of *Candida* infected saliva at the angles of the mouth where there is erythema, crusting and cracking. It is a general sign of candidiasis and may indicate systemic disorders including HIV infection and diabetes mellitus. Bacteria such as *S. aureus*, *E. coli* and *Pseudomonas* may also play a role in maintenance of the labial lesion.

Gingivitis and periodontal disease

Forms of gingivitis that involve acute inflammation with ulceration, which are promoted by heavy cigarette smoking or immunosuppression, often contain *Candida*, enteric bacteria and staphylococci. In addition, in persistant root canal infections, *C. albicans* is frequently isolated with oral streptococci, to which it can adhere (Figure 33.2), and with *Peptostreptococcus* and *Fusobacterium*.

Prosthetic implants

Infectious failures of dental implants are associated with complex microbial etiologies (see Chapter 28). After prolonged use of systemic antibacterial agents, or chlorhexidine mouth rinses, overgrowth of atypical periodontal organisms such as *C. albicans*, *S. aureus* and *Pseudomonas* may occur. In patients with surgical laryngectomies, a voice prosthesis acts as a shut valve between the trachea and esophagus. The medical-grade silicone rubber within the voice prosthesis are subject to microbial colonization. Mixed species biofilms comprising mainly of *Candida*, staphylococci, oral streptococci and enterococci form on the esophageal side, causing the valve mechanism to malfunction and the prosthesis fails. Central venous catheters, endotracheal tubes and urinary catheters become colonized by a range of microbes, and *Candida* species often feature in these polymicrobial infections.

Biofilms and antifungal drugs

Candida biofilms (Figure 33.3) are more resistant to antifungal compounds, including amphotericin B, fluconazole and nystatin, as well as to chlorhexidine. The reasons for this are still not entirely clear, but several genes encoding anti-fungal drug export pumps are up-regulated in biofilms. Recently, it has been shown that adherence initiates production of multi-drug tolerant persister cells within *C. albicans* biofilms. These slowly metabolizing or dormant cells probably confer reduced susceptibility to antifungal agents. This explains why *Candida* infections often cannot be eliminated with current antifungal drugs. The search for new antifungal agents has led to the discovery of echinocandins, such as caspofungin, that attack the glucan components of the *Candida* cell wall. Because of low bioavailability, echinocandins are given intravenously.

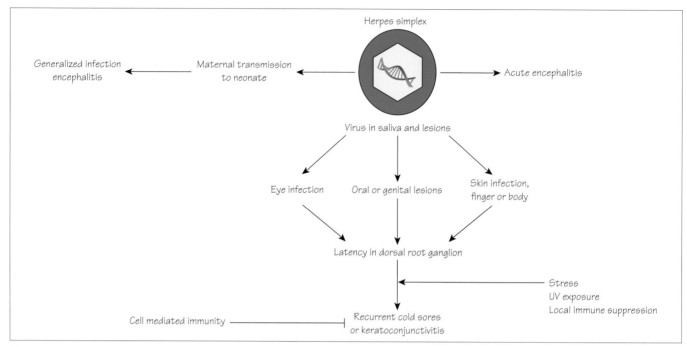

Figure 34.1 Progression and manifestations of herpes simplex infection.

Table 34.1 Characteristics of human herpes viruses.

Name	Common designation	Major disease(s)	Site of Latency	Transmission
HHV1	Herpes simplex 1	Stomatitis (cold sores) on oral epithelium	Neuron	Close contact, saliva
HHV2	Herpes simplex 2	Genital lesions	Neuron	Sexual and close contact
HHV3	Varicella zoster (VZV)	Chickenpox, shingles (after reactivation)	Neuron	Respiratory and close contact
HHV4	Epstein Barr (EBV)	Infectious mononucleosis, B-cell lymphomas, hairy oral leukoplakia	B-cell	Saliva
HHV5	Cytomegalovirus (CMV)	Congenital defects, opportunistic in immunocompromised patients	Monocyte, lymphocyte	Close contact, transfusion, congenital
HHV6	Herpes lymphotropic virus	Exanthema subitum (roseola or sixth disease)	T-cell	Respiratory, saliva and close contact
HHV7	Human herpesvirus 7	Unknown	T-cell	Unknown
HHV8	Kaposi's sarcoma-associated herpes virus (KSHV)	Kaposi's sarcoma, primary effusion lymphoma (PEL) and multicentric Castelman's disease (MCD)	Lymphocyte	Sexual, saliva, close contact

Many viruses can be acquired by mouth and are present in whole saliva. Viruses can also be present in the oral cavity following spread from other tissues. Herpes viruses, hepatitis B virus, rubella virus, measles virus, mumps virus and respiratory viruses such as influenza can all be spread by aerosols. Dentists are therefore at risk both of contracting viral infections and spreading viral infections among patients. In the next two chapters we shall discuss those viruses with most significance to dentistry.

Herpes viruses

Herpes viruses are large (150–200 nm), enveloped, icosahedral viruses containing double stranded linear DNA that replicate in the host cell nucleus. Herpes viruses can establish latency and cause persistent infections (Table 34.1).

(1) Herpes simplex virus 1 and 2 (HSV-1, HSV-2; human herpes virus 1, human herpes virus 2) (Figure 34.1)

HSV-1 is transmitted by contact with saliva and is usually acquired in early childhood. Primary infection is often asymptomatic, but bilateral stomatitis in the epithelium of the oral mucosa can occur for 2–3 weeks. Following primary infection, HSV-1 is transported up the trigeminal ganglia where it remains latent. Reactivation (brought about by stress, UV exposure, local immune suppression), results in transport of the virus back down the axon where infection and replication in epithelial cells occurs, causing unilateral stomatitis (cold sores).

The closely related HSV-2 virus is usually sexually transmitted and causes lesions in the genital area. However, HSV-2 can also cause disease in the oral cavity. Other sites of infections for HSV viruses include the throat (pharyngitis), eye (keratitis), finger (whitlow), and body (gladiatorum). In rare cases, usually associated with immune suppression, both HSV-1 and -2 can cause severe and fatal encephalitis.

TH-1 associated delayed type hypersensitivity cytotoxic T-cells are necessary to kill infected cells. Both HSV-1 and -2 can be treated with acyclovir, a drug that is activated by HSV thymidine kinase and blocks viral DNA polymerase.

(2) Varicella zoster virus (VZV, human herpes virus 3)

VZV causes varicella (chickenpox), after which virus becomes latent in ganglia along the entire neuraxis. Virus reactivation produces zoster (shingles). The virus is present in saliva and is spread by respiratory droplet and by direct contact.

(3) Epstein Barr virus (EBV, human herpes virus 4)

EBV is transmitted in saliva, and infection usually occurs in early childhood when it is asymptomatic. In later life, primary infection can cause infectious mononucleosis ('mono', kissing disease) with fever, swollen adenoid glands and fatigue. This disease is usually benign and self-limiting. EBV replicates primarily in B-cells and can cause B-cell transformation. EBV is thus associated with B-cell lymphomas such as Burkitt's lymphoma in Africa. EBV also infects epithelial cells and is associated with nasopharyngeal lymphoma in China. Hairy oral leukoplakia, that occurs mainly in AIDS patients, is a manifestation of EBV infection of epithelial cells in the oral cavity. EBV can remain latent in B-cells. T-cells are required for controlling infection.

(4) Cytomegalovirus (CMV, human herpes virus 5)

CMV infections can be spread by saliva and are usually asymptomatic, but primary infection in early pregnancy can lead to severe complications for the fetus. In immunocompromised (diminished cell-mediated immunity) patients, more severe symptoms occur such as retinitis, hepatitis and encephalitis. CMV infects many lymphocyte types, including macrophages. The virus can remain latent in lymphocytes and in tissue, and infected tissues show a characteristic 'owl's-eye' nuclear inclusion body.

(5) Human herpes viruses 6, 7 and 8 (HHV6, HHV7, HHV8)

HHV6 is associated with a common childhood disease, exanthema subitum (roseola, sixth disease). The virus replicates in the salivary glands and is secreted into saliva. Most infections are subclinical, and almost all adults are seropositive. HHV7 is detected in saliva but as yet has no known disease association. HHV8 is present in the saliva and is associated with the etiology of Kaposi's sarcoma.

Papillomaviruses

Papillomaviruses are small (50–55 nm) icosahedral, non-enveloped viruses containing double stranded DNA. They are members of the papovavirus family. Human papillomaviruses (HPV) cause warts on the skin and mucosal surfaces, including the oral soft tissues. There are several types of HPV that are based on DNA homology and these have different tropisms for epithelial cells. Some HPV possess oncogenes such as the E6 and E7 proteins of HPV-16 and HPV-18 that can cause cervical carcinoma and are also linked to oral cancer. HPV-6 and HPV-11 are associated with benign head and neck tumors.

Parvoviruses

Only one parvovirus, B19, is associated with human disease. B19 causes erythema infectiosum (fifth disease, slapped cheek syndrome) in children. In adults with sickle-cell disease or similar types of chronic anemia, B19 can cause an acute, severe anemia. B19 can also cause abortion if infection occurs during pregnancy. Parvoviruses are small (18–26 nm in diameter) with a non-enveloped icosahedral capsid. B19 has one linear, single strand DNA. Large numbers of virus are released into saliva.

Oral virology II, hepatitis and HIV

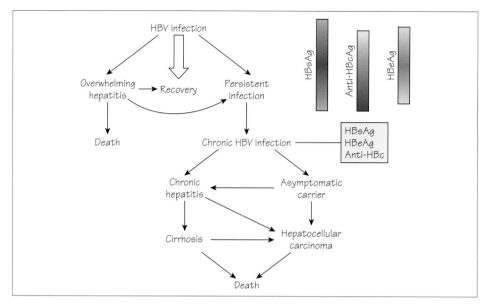

Figure 35.1 Outcomes of HBV infection and concentration changes in HBV antigens and antibodies.

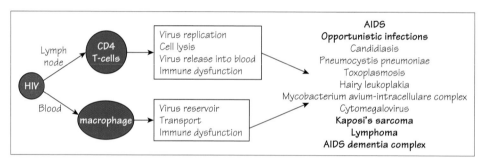

Figure 35.2 Major pathogenic mechanisms of human immunodeficiency virus (HIV) and disease outcomes.

Table 35.1 Vaccines against Hepatitis viruses

Vaccine and duration	Recommendations
Hepatitis A	Recommended for all children over one year
Inactivated virus	People age 12 months or older who are traveling to or working in areas of the world where Hepatitis A is endemic, or there is a known outbreak (fecal to oral transmission, usually by water). Vaccine or IgG to the virus can be given when exposure is suspected. Infants under 12 months can also receive IgG
Two dose series protects for at least 20 years in adults	People whose sexual activity puts them at risk
	People receiving clotting factor concentrates
Hepatitis B	Recommended for all newborns in many countries
Recombinant Surface	Health care workers, and research laboratory staff and students working with human tissues e.g. blood, saliva
Antigen S component	People exposed to blood contaminated body fluids through work, drug use or sexual activity
Three dose series protects for at least 20 years	Babies born to mothers with active hepatitis B infections. IgG to the virus should also be given
Hepatitis C	No current vaccine although promising future with development of a new animal model of infection
Hepatitis D Hepatitis B Vaccine	Not possible to acquire Hepatitis D unless subject already has Hepatitis B. Therefore, most effective approach against Hepatitis D is to get the Hepatitis B vaccine
Hepatitis E	Vaccine close to production. Will be recommended for travelers to sub-Saharan Africa, Central America, India and SE Asia (fecal to oral transmission, usually by water).

Hepatitis B virus (HBV)

HBV is a small (42 nm) enveloped virus, and a member of the hepadnavirus family. Genetic material is circular, partially double-stranded DNA. However, the virus produces a reverse transcriptase and replicates through an RNA intermediate. Surrounding the DNA and enzymes is the core antigen (HBcAg) and an envelope containing the surface antigen (HBsAg). HBeAg is related to HBcAg and is a minor component of the virion (Dane) particles, but is secreted into the serum. HBsAg is also secreted in filamentous (Australia antigen) or spherical particles. HBsAg includes three glycoproteins (L, M and S) encoded by the same gene but translated from different start codons.

HBV is transmitted by contact with contaminated blood and other human fluids such as saliva. The virus targets hepatocytes in the liver, and disease can be symptomatic or asymptomatic, and acute or chronic. The incubation period is about 2–6 months when inflammation of the liver, usually without high fever, occurs. During the latter half of the incubation period very high numbers of virions and surface antigen particles are present in the blood, and blood and saliva become infectious. The acute phase lasts about two months and then the numbers of virions and HBsAg particles drop, and antibodies to the core antigen develop. Antibodies to HBsAg do not develop until a number of weeks after the surface antigen is no longer detectable in the blood, but they can persist for several years. About 30% of infections are subclinical. In 10% of cases in adults, but up to 95% in neonates following vertical transmission, a chronic carrier state develops, with continued viral replication and no obvious symptoms. Of these, about 2% die of cirrhosis and 0.5% die of primary hepatocellular carcinoma (Figure 35.1).

Detection of HbsAg and HBeAg indicates active viral replication. Chronic infection can be distinguished by the continued presence of these antigens in the absence of detectable antibody. A vaccine for HBV comprises recombinant HBsAg S component (Table 35.1).

Hepatitis D virus (HDV, delta agent)

HDV is a defective virus that requires HBV to replicate. HDV has a small RNA genome surrounded by a delta antigen core and an HBsAg envelope. The requirement for HbsAg means that HDV either co-infects with HBV or superinfects chronic HBV carriers. In either case a fulminant hepatitis with high mortality is likely to occur.

Other hepatitis viruses

These are of less concern in a dental context. Hepatitis A (HAV, a picornavirus) and hepatitis E virus (HEV, a calcivirus) are spread by the fecal-oral route. HEV is more common in developing countries and can cause a fulminant hepatitis in pregnant women. Hepatitis C (HCV) and Hepatitis G (HGV) are flaviviruses that are transmitted through contaminated blood. HCV was a major cause of transfusion hepatitis before routine screening of donated blood. There is a possible association of hepatitis C with Sjögren's syndrome and with lichen planus.

Human immunodeficiency virus (HIV)

HIV is a member of the retrovirus family that are enveloped (80–120 nm in diameter) and contain two copies of positive strand RNA. Retroviruses encode an RNA-dependent DNA polymerase (reverse transcriptase) and thus replicate through a DNA intermediate that is integrated into the host cell chromosome. The HIV reverse transcriptase lacks proof reading capabilities and so the mutation rate for HIV is high, which contributes to immune avoidance and resistance to therapeutic agents (see below). HIV mainly infects cells expressing CD4 such as T helper cells, macrophages, dendritic cells and some neural glia cells. Co-receptors such as CXCR4 on T-cells and CCR5 on macrophages are also important for binding and infection. HIV causes proliferation and lysis of T-cells resulting in immune suppression, and there is also a persistent low level infection of macrophages. Immune suppression increases susceptibility to secondary infections and to tumor proliferation. In the oral cavity, HIV infection is associated with oral candidiasis (thrush), necrotizing ulcerative gingivitis (NUG) and hairy oral leukoplakia (Figure 35.2). HIV is present in body fluids such as blood, vaginal secretions and semen, however, transmission by saliva has not been demonstrated, possibly because of the anti-viral activity of some salivary molecules (Chapter 7).

Several treatment options are now available for HIV/AIDS. Reverse transcriptase inhibitors can be nucleoside analogs such as AZT, which are activated by phosphorylation, or non-nucleoside such as nevirapine. Protease inhibitors such as indinavir, block cleavage of the gag and gag-pol polyproteins which prevents virion morphogenesis. Current therapy calls for a cocktail of drugs with different mechanisms of action, termed highly active antiretroviral treatment (HAART).

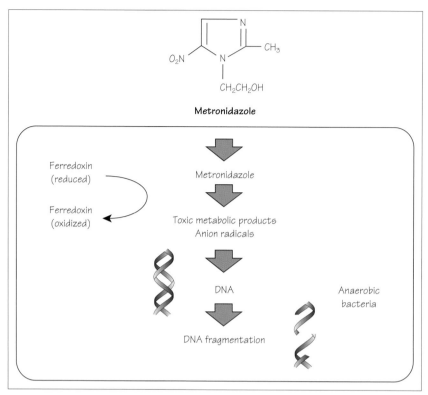

Figure 36.1 Mechanism of action of metronidazole.

Table 36.1 List of commonly-used antibiotics in clinical practice, their modes of action and some usually susceptible organisms.

Antibiotic	Principal mode of action	Susceptible organisms
Penicillin G and V, ampicillin, amoxicillin, cloxacillin	Cell wall biosynthesis (peptide cross-linking)	Streptococcus, Neisseria, Actinomyces
Augmentin	Cell wall biosynthesis (contains β-lactamase inhibitor)	Neisseria, Clostridium
Cephalosporins (cefotaxime)	Cell wall biosynthesis (peptide cross-linking)	Gram-negatives
Cycloserine	Cell wall biosynthesis (analog of D-alanine)	Staphylococcus, Mycobacterium
Vancomycin	Cell wall biosynthesis (peptidoglycan backbone)	Gram-positives
Aminoglycosides (streptomycin, gentamicin, kanamycin)	Protein synthesis (30S sub-unit detachment)	Gram-negatives Enterobacteriacae, Shigella
Tetracyclines (minocycline, doxycycline)	Protein synthesis (30S sub-unit tRNA acceptor site)	Haemophilus, Chlamydia, Bacteroides
Macrolides (erythromycin)	Protein synthesis (translocation)	Streptococcus, Gram-positives bacteria
Lincomycin, clindamycin	Protein synthesis (bind to 50S ribosomal sub-unit)	Gram-positives
Chloramphenicol	Protein synthesis	Neisseria, Enterococcus
Nitroimidazoles (metronidazole)	Nucleic acid synthesis (converted to compound that disrupts DNA helix)	Anaerobic bacteria

Antibiotic refers to any substance naturally produced by a microorganism that is inhibitory for another. It now also includes synthetic compounds that are antibacterial. Substances that kill sensitive organisms are bactericidal, while those that inhibit growth are bacteriostatic. The latter therefore rely on the host immune system to actually kill the infectious organism. Many bacterial species that were previously sensitive to antibiotics have acquired resistance (or reduced sensitivity). The important factor in this is the selection pressure imposed by antibiotic usage for less antibiotic-sensitive organisms. It is generally agreed, therefore, that unnecessary usage of antibiotics only fuels the development of antibiotic resistance. Although many antibiotics are taken orally, the levels of antibiotics such as penicillins and erythromycin present in saliva are much less than those achieved in serum. The reverse is true for the macrolide azithromycin. Commonly-used antibiotics are described in Table 36.1.

Antibiotics in dentistry

The most commonly prescribed antibiotics in dentistry are β-lactams (penicillins and cephalosporins), clindamycin, tetracyclines (especially local delivery in periodontal disease) and metronidazaole. Production of β-lactamases, which destroy penicillins and some cephalosporins, by streptococci is very rare. Hence streptococci generally have retained sensitivity to amoxicillin, and this is a frontline antibiotic administered by dental clinicians. However, levels of resistance are increasing amongst α-hemolytic streptococci, e.g. *S. pneumoniae*, and interspecies transfer of resistance determinants by DNA-mediated transformation is of major concern. Resistance is determined by mutations in a penicillin-binding protein (PBP2B) such that enzymic activity in cell wall biogenesis is unaffected by the antibiotic. Generally bacteria such as *P. gingivalis* remain relatively penicillin sensitive. However, in one study about 30% of *F. nucleatum* isolated from odontogenic infections were shown to produce β-lactamase enzymes. In view of this, there are recommendations for using clindamycin (active against most Gram-positives and Gram-negative anaerobes) in endodontic infections. Clindamycin is also the first-line agent in patients with penicillin allergy, but can cause antibiotic-associated colitis. Metronidazole, which also inhibits anaerobic bacteria, is particularly useful in periodontal disease (Figure 36.1). Emergence of resistance is not of major concern at the moment, partly because metronidazole is often used in combination with another antibiotic in order to counteract less anaerobic organisms. However, increasing resistance to metronidazole amongst *Helicobacter pylori* isolates is evident.

Resistance to anti-microbial agents

S. pneumoniae, and enterococci isolated from root canal infections, show high levels of resistance to cephalosporins. Cefotaxime resistance is easily transferred across α-hemolytic streptococci. The general level of resistance in the oral microbiota is not clear, but the potential for commensal bacteria to pass resistance on to more pathogenic species is of concern. A relatively high incidence of resistance to tetracycline is found in the oral microbiota. Up to 50% of oral isolates have been found to carry one or more of the tet resistance genes that confer resistance by ribosomal protection, tetracycline efflux, enzymatic inactivation, or modification of the ribosomal target. Often tetracycline resistance is linked with genes encoding penicillin, vancomycin or erythromycin resistance on the same transposable element. Tetracyclines are now used less frequently in dental practice because of the side effects of these drugs, one of which is to affect tooth color.

Transfer of anti-microbial resistance

Antibiotic resistance determinants can be spread by transformation and conjugation, and can be carried on transposons and integrons. Conjugation of plasmids and conjugative transposition can result in acquisition of multiple drug resistance genes. Oral microbial biofilms provide a means for microbes to exist in close proximity, facilitating genetic exchange between the bacteria by conjugative plasmids or by conjugative transposons. For example, high transfer frequencies of tetM, by a Tn916-like element, between *Veillonella* and *Streptococcus* have been found. These organisms grow together in an inter-nutritional relationship (Chapter 14). There is also concern about the increasingly high prevalence of antibiotic resistance genes within ingested bacteria, especially probiotic preparations. Organisms in foods carrying antimicrobial resistance determinants have the potential to transfer those determinants to the oral microbiota.

Curtailing anti-microbial resistance

New guidelines in the UK and USA do not recommend prophylatic administration of antibiotics as coverage for dental procedures in most patients. This represents a major effort to reduce what is considered the unnecessary usage of antibiotics. New antibacterial approaches, such as biomimetics for inhibition of biofilm development, natural plant products and biological interference, provide alternatives to antibiotic usage. These may help contain the development and spread of antibiotic resistant organisms. A major future challenge will be to identify potential antibiotic resistance determinants within the ~50% oral bacterial species that have not yet been cultivated. This may reveal new resistance genes for current antibiotics, as well as possibly new anti-microbials.

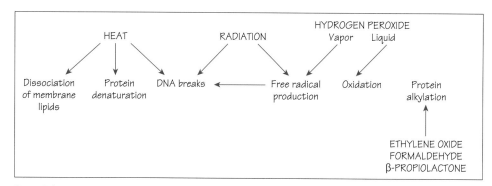

Figure 37.1 Mode of action of the major sterilization agents.

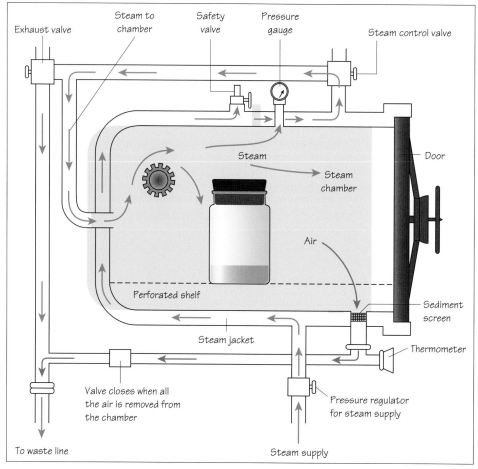

Figure 37.2 Moist heat sterilization in an autoclave.

Sterilization is the complete elimination of all forms of life, whereas disinfection is the reduction or removal of potential infectivity. Antisepsis refers to disinfection of living tissues. The mode of action of common sterilizing agents is shown in Figure 37.1.

Heat

Heat kills by denaturation of proteins, causing single strand breaks in DNA and dissociation of membrane lipids. Vegetative cells of bacteria, fungi and viruses are killed within a few minutes at 60–80°C. However, bacterial spores are more resistant to heat and sterilization requires temperatures over 120°C.

(1) Moist heat Steam is heated to 121–132°C by applying a pressure of 104 kPa (15 lb/in^2). Sterilization requires at least 15 minutes. Moist heat sterilization is accomplished in an autoclave (Figure 37.2). Parameters such as load/chamber volume ratio and flow rate of steam affect the time required for killing. It is important that no air pockets remain in the autoclave chamber as these prevent penetration of the steam. The temperature can be monitored with a thermocouple, and autoclave tape is useful to distinguish autoclaved from non-autoclaved material. However, biological effectiveness of sterilization should be monitored with a spore test. A strip or vial of *Bacillus stearothermophilus* spores is placed in the center of the load and tested for subsequent failure to germinate. Most instruments can be sterilized by autoclaving, although some metals corrode. Paper and other non-wettables cannot be autoclaved.

(2) Dry heat Hot air is heated at 160–180°C for 1–2 hours. This is not as efficient as moist heat as penetration of air is slower than steam, and lack of water makes hydrogen bonds more stable and reduces the rate of protein denaturation. Dry heat ovens are useful for materials that are damaged by water. Killing should be tested with spores of *Bacillus subtilis* which are more resistant to dry heat than spores of *B. stearothermophilus*.

Radiation

Ionizing radiation from X-rays or γ-rays with wavelengths less than 200 nm break chemical bonds and ionize molecules. Free radicals then cause damage to DNA. Radiation requires expensive equipment and shielding, so is more commonly used by commercial suppliers of disposables.

Chemicals

(1) Ethylene oxide This is an alkylating gas (transfers a CH_3 group) that causes protein denaturation. It does not require water for activity, but sterilization takes over three hours' exposure. It can be used on wrapped surgical materials such as sponges and plastics that cannot be sterilized by heat. Sterilized material should not be handled for at least 24 hours to allow any residual ethylene oxide to evaporate.

(2) Formaldehyde This is an alkylating agent. It is only effective over a narrow concentration range. A residue of pararformaldehyde can form on surfaces, which depolymerizes to formaldehyde and irritates the skin.

(3) Hydrogen peroxide At concentrations of 10–25% hydrogen peroxide is sterilizing. A more recent innovation is plasma gas sterilization using vaporized hydrogen peroxide. Radio-frequency energy is applied to create an electric field, which transforms the hydrogen peroxide vapor into a low-temperature gas plasma and generates free radicals.

(4) β-propiolactone This alkylating gas is very toxic to humans and rarely used.

(5) Chemical vapor (chemiclave) This uses a combination of formaldehyde, alcohols, acetone, ketones and steam at 138–176 kPa and 127–132°C for 30 minutes. It is useful in the dental setting as it does not corrode instruments or destroy heat sensitive materials, and is faster than dry heat sterilization. Adequate ventilation must be available to remove fumes released when the chamber is opened.

38 Disinfection

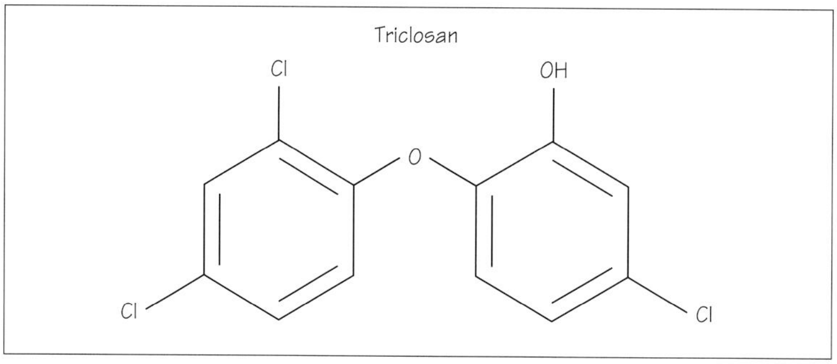

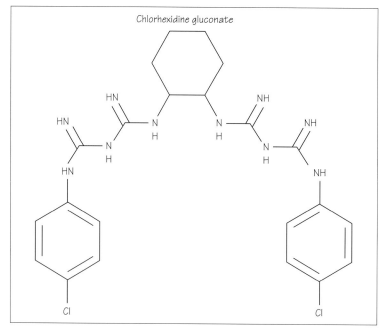

Figure 38.1 Structure of triclosan.

Figure 38.2 Structure of chlorhexidine.

Table 38.1 Common disinfectants and their principal mode of action.

Agent	Principal mode of action
UV light	Thymidine dimers in DNA
Laser light	Photothermal
Ultrasound	Cavitation waves
Phenols	Membrane disruption and protein denaturation
Halogens	Oxidation
Alcohols	Membrane disruption and protein denaturation
Aldehydes	Protein denaturation by alkyaltion
Surfactants	Membrane disruption
Diguanides	Membrane disruption
Oxidants	Oxidation, free radical generation and protein denaturation

The optimal disinfecting agent depends on the types of organism present, the physical nature of the material to be treated, and the amount of organic matter present. Common disinfectants are described in Table 38.1.

Physical

(1) Filtration This is useful for liquids. Pore size filters 0.22–0.45 μm remove most bacteria and fungi. Filtration does not remove viruses, mycoplasma and some small bacteria.

(2) Ultraviolet (UV) light Maximal killing by UV light occurs at 260 nm, the wavelength optimally absorbed by nucleic acids. UV light induces the formation of dimers between adjacent pyrimidine bases which block the progress of DNA and RNA polymerases. In addition, repair systems are activated, some of which are error prone and introduce mutations. The disadvantage of UV light is that it is poorly penetrating. UV light is produced by mercury vapor lamps which are used for control of airborne contamination or to disinfect surfaces when people are absent.

(3) Laser light Nd:YAG, Er:YAG, Er,Cr:YSGG, diode and KTP lasers can be used for photothermal disinfection, including in root canals, carious lesions and periodontal pockets. In addition, bacteria can be photosensitized with compounds such as tolonium chloride, toluidine blue or aluminum disulfonated phthalocyanine, and killed with low power lasers such as helium/neon or gallium aluminum arsenide lasers, by a photochemical reaction that produces reactive oxygen species, a technique termed photo-activated disinfection (PAD). Photodynamic therapy using PAD is less likely to damage host tissues.

(4) Ultrasound and sound Ultrasonic (and upper audible) waves with frequencies greater than 20 kHz will kill microorganisms. Sound waves in liquid produce cavitations which collapse violently and physically disrupt cell structures. Bacteria vary greatly in susceptibility; however, organic material is readily dislodged from contaminated surfaces. Sonic toothbrushes use sound waves around 6 kHz that create waves of pressure and shear forces that help dislodge plaque, along with cavitation waves. The long-term effects of these on host tissues are unknown.

Chemical

(1) Phenol-based compounds Phenol kills organisms primarily by disrupting lipid containing membranes, and hence is poorly active against spores and non-enveloped viruses. However phenolic compounds are active against mycobacteria due to the high lipid content of mycobacterial cell walls, and phenols are not easily inactivated by organic matter. Activity can be increased by emulsifying in detergent to improve solubility and penetration. In addition, substituting the organic ring with a halogen, alkyl or hydroxyl group increases activity, and two linked phenols (bis-phenols or diphenyls) are more active. Triclosan is a halogenated phenolic used in toothpastes and in plastics as a surface

antimicrobial (Figure 38.1). Triclosan is also used as a skin disinfectant to control methicillin resistant *S. aureus*. Other examples of phenolics are Lysol and chloroxylenol (Dettol).

(2) Halogens Compounds based on iodine or chlorine are very effective disinfectants. Iodine combines irreversibly with some amino acids and is also an oxidant. It is useful for disinfecting skin or mucus membranes prior to surgery. Iodine is most active at pH less than 6, and kills most bacteria (including mycobacteria), viruses, and even shows some activity against bacterial spores. Iodine can be dissolved in alcohol (tincture) or complexed with a carrier such as a detergent (iodophor). Povidone iodine (iodine complexed with polyvinylpyrrolidone) is commonly used. Some individuals are allergic. Examples are Wescodyne and Betadine. Chlorine is generally used as a 5% solution of sodium hypochlorite. Chlorine is a strong oxidizing agent that is active against vegetative bacteria and viruses. Organic matter and alkaline detergents reduce effectiveness. Sodium hypochlorite is often used as an irrigant in root canal therapy. An example is Chlorox.

(3) Alcohols These disrupt lipid membranes and denature proteins. Activity is improved in aqueous solutions of about 70%, and activity increases with chain length, up to eight carbons when insolubility becomes a problem. Alcohols kill vegetative bacteria, some fungi and enveloped viruses. They are easily inactivated by organic matter. Ethanol (C2) and isopropanol (C3) are the most common.

(4) Aldehydes Glutaraldehyde is commonly used as a disinfectant although it is toxic to living tissues. Glutaraldehyde is optimally active at pH 8.5 which is attained by "activation" with sodium hydroxide/bicarbonate. Glutaraldehyde alkylates and denatures proteins and is active against most bacteria and viruses, and shows some activity against spores. Glutaraldehyde is easily inactivated by organic matter.

(5) Surface active agents (surfactants) These are compounds that contain both hydrophobic and hydrophilic regions and can thus solubilize lipid membranes. Among the more effective are the cationic quaternary ammonium compounds such as benzalkonium chloride, with four organic groups covalently linked to nitrogen. Activity is greatest against Gram-positives. They are easily inactivated by organic matter.

(6) Diguanides Chlorhexidine is used in mouthwash (at 0.2%, e.g. Peridex) for plaque control and at higher concentrations (2%) as a denture disinfectant (Figure 38.2). An advantage of chlorhexidine is the property of substantivity, whereby the compound binds to oral surfaces and remains active over extended time periods. Chlorhexidine is deactivated by anionic compounds, including SDS, commonly used as detergents in toothpastes. Thus, chlorhexidine mouth rinses should be used at least 30 minutes after other dental products. Chlorhexidine is active against bacteria (but not mycobacteria) and *Candida*, but is easily inactivated by organic matter.

(7) Oxidizing agents Hydrogen peroxide (3%) and potassium permanganate (1%) oxidize proteins and other cellular constituents and generate free radicals.

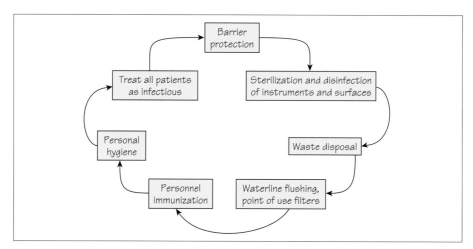

Figure 39.1 *Major components of an effective infection control policy.*

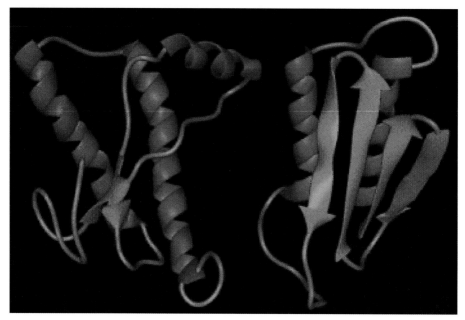

Figure 39.2 Prions. Normal prion protein (left) can change its own conformation to the misfolded infectious prion (right), and induce other prions to become abnormally folded. The misfolded prions aggregate into an amyloid structure containing densely packed beta-sheets, and damage tissues.

Infection control in the dental setting is designed to prevent transmission of infectious disease and is based on the assumption that *all patients are potentially infectious.*

There are several elements to an effective, universal infection control policy (Figure 39.1).

(1) Patient evaluation Medical history should be recorded and updated on each visit. This will reveal specific infectious diseases.

(2) Personal hygiene Hands should be washed with liquid anti-microbial soap. Open wounds should be covered. Hair should be short or tied up. Fingernails should be trimmed and jewelry should be removed.

(3) Personal protection Disposable covers should be placed on frequently handled surfaces. New gloves should be worn for each patient. Sterile gloves should be worn for surgical procedures. Heavy duty gloves should be worn when cleaning instruments. Gowns should be worn and changed at least daily. Eye shields and facemasks should be worn. A rubber dam should be used to isolate the tooth and minimize aerosol and splatter when appropriate. Sharps should be discarded in a puncture resistant sharps container.

(4) Sterilization and disinfection Instruments, materials and surfaces should be sterilized or disinfected as discussed in Chapters 37 and 38. Disposal of all clinical waste should follow local guidelines.

(5) Immunization Dental health care personnel should be immunized against hepatitis B, measles-mumps-rubella, varicella-zoster, polio, diphtheria-tetanus-pertussis and influenza (annually). In some countries the BCG vaccine against tuberculosis is recommended. A hepatitis A vaccine is available, but is not specifically recommended for dental personnel.

Prions

Prions are isoforms of a normal protein and are capable of self-propagation although they lack nucleic acid (Figure 39.2). Prion diseases have an incubation period of years and are usually fatal within one year of diagnosis. In humans, prions cause progressively fatal transmissible spongiform encephalopathies (TSEs) including kuru, Creutzfeldt-Jakob disease (CJD), and variant CJD (vCJD). There is no evidence linking dental procedures to infection with TSEs. However, such an association cannot be completely excluded. Moreover, prions are exceptionally resistant to physical and chemical sterilization. It is probably wise, therefore, when treating a patient with known prion disease to employ single-use instruments which are then incinerated, as far as is practicable. Disinfectants that can reduce the infectivity of prions include chlorine, guanidine thiocyanate and sodium hydroxide. Sterilization may require 121–132°C for 60 minutes or longer. Autoclaving at 134–138°C for 18 minutes or in six three-minute cycles followed by immersion in sodium hydroxide (2 M) or sodium hypochloride (20,000 ppm) has also been recommended.

Dental unit water lines (DUWL)

Biofilms form readily on the inside surfaces of DUWL. Bacteria can be shed from these biofilms and released in aerosols. Most of the bacteria in these biofilms are harmless (in immunocompetent individuals) environmental organisms, originating from the water source. However, opportunistic respiratory pathogens such as *Pseudomomas aeruginosa*, mycobacteria and *Legionella* have also been detected, as have oral bacteria that presumably originate from backflow from dental apparatus. While the risk of disease from bacteria in DUWL is small, American Dental Association guidelines are that water from DUWL contains fewer than 200 cfu/ml. To achieve these levels, DUWL should be flushed for two minutes at the beginning of each day and for 30 seconds between patients. DUWL should also have independent water reservoirs and be fitted with point of use filters to prevent backflow.

40 Bioterrorism

Table 40.1 Highly infectious or pathogenic microorganisms that have been considered bioterrorism agents, the diseases and symptoms, exposure and dosage, and treatment or prevention.

Agent	Disease	Transmission	Exposure	Infectious dose	Incubation/onset	Symptoms	Treatment and prevention
Bacterial							
Bacillus anthracis	Anthrax	Infected animal tissue	Skin	Unknown	2–5 days	Cutaneous: insect bite-like mark developing into blister/skin necrosis. Fever and headache	Numerous effective antibiotics available (intravenously for inhalational anthrax)
		Contaminated soil, animal hides	Inhalation	2.5–50 k cells		Inhalational: sore throat, fever, difficulty breathing, shock/meningitis or pneumonia	Vaccine available to high risk workers
		Contaminated undercooked meat	Ingestion	Unknown		Gastrointestinal: sore throat, loss of appetite, vomiting/fever, fluid filled abdomen – shock/death	
Yersinia pestis	Plague (pneumonic, bubonic, septicemic)	Exposure to infected animals	Inhalation	100–20,000 cells	Pneumonic: 2–4 days	Pneumonic: severe cough, bloody sputum, difficulty breathing	Antibiotics available, must be given within first 24 hours of infection
					Bubonic: 1–8 days	Bubonic: fever/malaise, buboes, headache, seizures	
		Flea bites	Skin	Unknown	Septicemic: 2–6 days post pneumonic or bubonic infection	Septicemic: abdominal pain, blood clotting problems, low blood pressure, vomiting, organ failure	Vaccine available to high risk workers
Francisella tularensis	Tularemia (pneumonic, ulceroglandular, oropharyngeal, typhoidal)	Contaminated dust	Inhalation	5–10 cells	3–5 days	Pneumonic: cough, chest pains, difficulty breathing	Effective antibiotics available
		Handling infected animals	Skin	10–50 cells		Ulceroglandular: ulcer at site of infection, swollen lymph glands, fever/chills, headache, exhaustion	Vaccine not currently available
		Arthropod bite				Oropharyngeal: vomiting	
		Contaminated food or water	Ingestion	10^6–10^8 cells		Typhoidal: (rare) fever, extreme exhaustion, weight loss	
Burkholderia pseudomallei	Melioidosis	Contaminated soil or water	Inhalation	Unknown	2–9 days	Pneumonic: fever, headache, chest pains, mild bronchitis to severe pneumonia	Numerous effective antibiotics available
		Handling infected animals	Skin			Cutaneous: abscess/ulcer at site of infection, regional lymphadenopathy	No vaccine
						Chronic infection may affect the heart, brain, liver, kidneys and eyes	
						Septicemia/bacteremia may occur in immunocompromised individuals	
Brucella spp.	Brucellosis	Contaminated meat/dairy products	Ingestion	Unknown	5–60 days	Undulant fever, chills, weight loss, headache, abdominal/back pain, swollen glands; can become chronic	Effective antibiotics available
			Inhalation (rare; mainly vets, slaughterhouse workers and lab workers)	10–100 cells			No human vaccine
		Handling infected animals	Skin	Unknown			
Toxins							
Clostridium botulinum toxin	Botulism (flaccid paralysis)	Food borne	Ingestion	Unknown in humans; estimated to be between 1.2–12 ng/kg	12–72 hrs by any route of exposure	Dysphagia, blurred/double vision, dry mouth, nausea, abdominal cramps, muscle weakness, difficulty breathing/respiratory failure, descending paralysis (flaccid paralysis)	Anti-toxin available
			Inhalation (in weaponised or aerosolised form)				May require surgical intervention
							Intensive care

Table 40.1 (Continued)

Agent	Disease	Transmission	Exposure	Infectious dose	Incubation/onset	Symptoms	Treatment and prevention
Clostridium perfringens (epsilon toxin)	Clostridial myonecrosis (gas gangrene)	Contaminated water or soil	Inoculation into open wounds	Undefined for humans	10–12 hrs (after ingestion of whole cells)	Gas gangrene: tachycardia, moderate/high fever, severe pain around site of injury/infection, blisters/air under skin, drainage from tissues; can result in shock and organ failure	Gas gangrene: intravenous antibiotics or surgical debridement
	Food poisoning	Food borne	Ingestion Inhalation (in weaponised or aerosolised form)		Onset following ingestion/inhalation of toxin is unknown	Food poisoning: vomiting and diarrhea	Food poisoning: self-limiting, usually not treated
Staphylococcal enterotoxin B	Food poisoning	Food borne	Ingestion Inhalation (in weaponised or aerosolised form)	Estimated to be 20 ng/kg	3–12 hrs by any route of exposure	Food poisoning: nausea, vomiting and diarrhea Inhalational: sudden onset of fever, chills, headache, non-productive cough, chest pain, respiratory distress, hypotension, shock/death	Food poisoning: self-limiting and not usually life-threatening.
Viral Orthopox virus (variola)	Smallpox	Person to person (virus is confined to human host only)	Inhalation Contact with skin lesions or secretions	Estimated to be 10–100 virions	10–17 days	High fever, fatigue, severe headache, backache, malaise, raised pink rash (pus-filled lesions; day 8–9) vomiting, diarrhea, excessive bleeding, delirium	Vaccinia based live vaccine available No effective anti-virals
Filoviruses (Ebola)	Hemorrhagic fever	Person to person (natural reservoir unknown)	Contact with infected blood, secretions or organs	Undefined for humans; less than ten virions for non-human primates	5–12 days	Fever, sore throat, weakness, severe headache, joint/muscle ache, vomiting, dehydration, dry cough, rash, liver and kidney failure, inability to clot/internal and external hemorrhage, death in second week of infection (intractable shock)	No vaccine No effective anti-virals
Arenaviruses (Lassa)	Hemorrhagic fever	Person to person Handling infected animals	Inhalation Skin	Unknown	7–21 days	Fever, chest pains, sore throat, back/abdominal pain, cough, vomiting and diarrhea, conjunctivitis, facial swelling, mucosal bleeding. Neurological symptoms may include hearing loss, tremors and encephalitis	No vaccine No effective anti-virals
Alphaviruses (Venezuelan equine encephalitis virus)	Encephalitis	Mosquito bite	Skin Inhalation (in weaponised or aerosolised form)	One virion	2–6 days	Low grade/moderate fever, headache/retro-orbital pain, nausea/vomiting, dehydration leading to hypotension, altered mental status, paralysis, coma	No vaccine No effective anti-virals

Biological agents (Table 40.1) have been used in war to incapacitate and kill for hundreds of years. An early recorded example in which biological warfare was employed dates back to the fourteenth century when during a conflict between Mongols and Italian traders the corpses of plague victims were catapulted into the city of Kaffa, resulting in a devastating outbreak of the plague. Similarly in 1763, following numerous hostilities between the British and Native Americans, smallpox-laced blankets were distributed to the Native Americans under the guise of a gesture of goodwill, leading to outbreaks of smallpox. The development and employment of biological weapons became more sophisticated and during both World Wars numerous bacterial, viral and toxin based weapons were developed and tested. This continued into the Cold War which saw extensive stockpiling of biological weapons, followed by the introduction of treaties to encourage disarmament.

Anthrax

The use of anthrax as a biological weapon emerged during the First World War, initially by Germany and later the UK, as a means of killing livestock and subsequently causing starvation. German agents planned anthrax and glanders attacks in a number of countries during World War I. World War II saw further development towards a weapon designed to incapacitate and kill humans. Extensive testing of anthrax bombs was carried out on Gruinard Island (off the coast of Scotland). *Bacillus anthracis* spores persisted in the soil for thirty years, after which time the land was decontaminated using a mixture of seawater and formaldehyde. In 2001, letters containing anthrax spores were delivered to news media offices and the US Congress, killing five people.

Botulism

Clostridium botulinum toxin was developed as a biological weapon over 60 years ago in Japan. During the Cold War years the USSR produced many thousands of liters of botulinum toxin, which was later destroyed as part of a disarmament program. The toxin can be produced in abundance and with relative ease; approximately 19,000 liters was produced by Iraq in the 1980s, much of which was incorporated into missiles and bombs. This amount is enough to kill the entire human population on earth.

Smallpox

Smallpox is regarded as the greatest threat if acquired by dissident organizations and used as a biological weapon. Only two repositories exist in the world, in Atlanta (USA) and Novosibirsk (Russia). If aerosolised, smallpox could easily be disseminated throughout a population and would spread rapidly from person to person. Worldwide reserves of the smallpox vaccine are limited, and during the 1970s when endemic smallpox was officially eradicated stringent vaccine programs were relaxed, meaning that there is a potentially vulnerable population.

Salmonella

Although not considered a significant bioterrorism agent, *Salmonella* was used in the first confirmed bioterrorism attack in the USA. In 1984, in an attempt to control local elections, followers of the Bhagwan Shree Rajneesh infected salad bars in The Dalles, Oregon, with *Salmonella enterica* Typhimurium. Over 700 people contracted food poisoning, but there were no fatalities.

Biological Weapons Convention

The Biological Weapons Convention was built upon the Geneva protocol of 1925, and was implemented in 1975. This prohibits the development, stockpiling and use of biological and toxin-based weapons. Initially 22 governments joined, and this number has risen in subsequent years. Consequently, numerous disarmament programs have been implemented worldwide.

Index

Note: page numbers with a 't' next to them refer to tables; page numbers with an 'f' next to them refer to figures.